This Watery Place

"A fierce and luminous revelation, *This Watery Place* proposes gestation as a common and necessary infrastructure of militancy. Written from the postpartum season's immense derangement of the senses, Heaney's thought carries across the rubble of the pandemic era, moving from gestation to the miracle of the newborn stranger, who, appearing everywhere, calls us to unmake and remake collective life. This is a work of total antagonism against the grim proposition that the cruelty of the present is the only possible world."
—Anne Boyer, poet and author of *The Undying*

"An astonishing achievement. This 'worker's inquiry' into the labor of gestation is written with the propulsiveness of a novel, the vulnerability of memoir, and the diagnostic precision of the best historical materialist analysis. I gasped at the brilliance of Heaney's argumentation more than once; and I often found myself wanting to stop and cry at the beauty of a particular sentence or paragraph. But I didn't stop, because the desire to know what new prismatic formulation would kaleidoscope into shape, pushed me on. If you have wondered whether a genuinely dialectical auto-theoretical project is possible, it is. Although maybe only Emma Heaney can write it."
—Jordy Rosenberg, author of *Confessions of the Fox*

"Quite simply the articulation of communism I have been waiting for. In theorizing the profound and universal freedom immanent to the hydraulics of provision, Heaney rescues gestation from pregnancy, and sets not only feminism but also Marxism on its feet. This book will be recognized as one of the major and most vital interventions of the decade."
—Sophie Lewis, author of *Abolish the Family*

This Watery Place

Four Essays on Gestation

Emma Heaney

First published 2025 by Pluto Press
New Wing, Somerset House, Strand, London WC2R 1LA
and Pluto Press, Inc.
1930 Village Center Circle, 3-834, Las Vegas, NV 89134

www.plutobooks.com

Copyright © Emma Heaney 2025

The right of Emma Heaney to be identified as the author of this work has been asserted in accordance with the Copyright, Designs and Patents Act 1988.

British Library Cataloguing in Publication Data
A catalogue record for this book is available from the British Library

ISBN 978 0 7453 5014 1 Paperback
ISBN 978 0 7453 5016 5 PDF
ISBN 978 0 7453 5015 8 EPUB

This book is printed on paper suitable for recycling and made from fully managed and sustained forest sources. Logging, pulping and manufacturing processes are expected to conform to the environmental standards of the country of origin.

Typeset by Stanford DTP Services, Northampton, England

Simultaneously printed in the United Kingdom and United States of America

EU GPSR Authorised Representative
LOGOS EUROPE, 9 rue Nicolas Poussin, 17000, LA ROCHELLE, France
Email: Contact@logoseurope.eu

J.E.H and N.H.H.:
from, with, for

Contents

Acknowledgments viii
Preface: Us xi

One: Fetal Separateness 1
Two: Is a Cervix Cis? 36
Three: The Hydraulics of Provision 61
Four: Wars, Wars, Wars; or Swimming in the Waters
of the World 91

Notes 122

Acknowledgments

Sophie Lewis's thought welcomed me to gestation and guided me through its seasons. Twice, in early labor in my apartment, pausing to time contractions, I packed my hospital bag with their books. Six hours postpartum in August 2021, I reread the "Amniotechnics" chapter of *Full Surrogacy Now* in the hospital bed to experience the difference between what had been and what was. In the same pose, twenty-one months later, I read the entirety of *Abolish the Family*, allowing my love to bloom like dye in the water of that book's utopian promise. I give thanks to the universe for Sophie's prism mind, which started this project. I thank them personally for the comradeship and interlocution that has sustained its creation.

David Shulman was this book's second champion and I'm so grateful for his interest, patience, and skill. Thanks also to the entire Pluto collective for holding down in general and for their work on this book. The anonymous readers of the proposal really helped. Many thanks to Dr. Autumn Womack who listened to my thinking toward "Is a Cervix Cis?" and brought the resulting essay to Angie Cruz, who published it in *Asterix Journal*, another origin of this volume.

To Lori, Nicole, and Stella: I'm so grateful for all your kind support that has made this book possible.

To my fellow-travelers: Marija Cetinic, M.E. O'Brien, Gabriel Foster, Greta La Fleur, Carla Macal Montenegro, Skira Martinez, Margaux Kristjansson, Juno Richards, Jules Gill-Peterson, Sumi Ragavan, Laura di Summa Knoop, Navyug Gill, Anupreet Sidhu, N—— Gill, S—— Gill, Laura Fisher, Colby Gordon, Travis Foster and family, Mustafa Saifuddin,

ACKNOWLEDGMENTS

Ms. Rachel, Julie Napolin, Amy Zanoni, R—— Zanoni, Jordy Rosenberg, Eva Heyward, Caitie Moore, Kira Josefsson, Jacqui Cornetta, Hannah Black, B—— Black, Katherine Quispe Garces, Adam Sanchez, D—— Sanchez Garces, Neeny Jenny, Michael, Gustavo, little O, baby F——, Sra. Ora, and Tangni: I love you and yours as mine. Thank you for being together at every stage.

Special thanks to Sophia Grady for being the quiet force in the house, for strings of drying persimmons, for a drink together in the evening. Thanks to Jess Braverman, Esquire for reviewing the law claims and for more than twenty years of steady friendship. To my ladies: Nada Ayad and Janet Neary, thank you for holding me up with your style and your thoughts. Thanks to Yuly Restrepo, my heart's writing friend.

To my brothers Noah, Forrest, and Sam, to Cousin N——, and my aunties Deb, Deb, Pam, Margy, and Barb: thank you for making the girls' lives full of love, aprons, books, and hand-knitted frog and toad dolls with tiny recreations of the clothes from M——'s favorite stories.

My girls' mamus and Khala: Sulman Afridi, Hasan Iqbal, Zara Afridi, and Simon Sandh, made a soft place for the babies to land; they keep remaking it.

Their Nanu, Mrs. Asma Afridi, has shown such care for me and such delighted devotion to the girls. What good fortune that someone so skilled in the intuitive art of loving patiently counted the beads of the abacus and taught my babies their first words.

From Cathy Murphy, the cultivator of herbs, flowers, children's souls, and public libraries, everything truly, and to her everything is due. My father, Eric Heaney, died when my first daughter was nine months old. His courage, his love, his small ways, and his insistence that his death be his death: all these are here in this book and in every day of my life.

With my co-parent and comrade Lena Afridi I learn to keep faith with the Quranic imperative to heed the ties of kinship.

Finally, to J—— and N——: I hope that the fidelity to life itself that each of you, in your singularity, has revived in me will redound on your lives for the good. Simply, to meet you every morning is the renewal of joy. To provide for you is my life's greatest privilege. I'm so grateful to be bound to you and like Morrison said, when you came, you brought me the most profound freedom. I hope to offer you a similar bond that frees. With gratitude to everyone and everything that sustains you, to you two together, this book is dedicated.

Preface: Us

This book was born in the postpartum ward. The on-duty nurse had come an hour previous to take my daughter for her first bath, which is performed at twenty-four hours of life to avoid chilling the baby upon their entry into the world of variable temperature. I'd been dozing off and on since the delivery at four a.m. the morning before. Now relieved from my first shift of a blessed vigilance, the duty to stare at my baby's chest to ensure the continuance of its minute rise and fall, I finally fell asleep.

I closed my eyes as they wheeled her away covered in the smell of oxidized iron; my dried blood — our shared blood — still lining the folds of her skin in a body net of deep oxblood red. When I opened my eyes again she'd been positioned six inches away from my face in the clear plastic hospital bassinet. She was scrubbed clean, arms swaddled tightly to her sides, wearing the familiar pink and blue striped hat, this one with a bow that stretched wider than her face. Her skin seemed to have gained substance in the interim that she'd been away. She was already losing some of the pearlescent quality of her neo-natalism born of nine and a half months growing in the liquid that had been circulating through us.

This availability of *us* as a singular pronoun was receding as the liquid indistinction between her body and mine waned. *Us* was regaining its grammatical coherence: it would once more mean you and me, or so it seemed in this first melancholy cognition of the rending. Although she was asleep, a blue pacifier bobbed in and out so vigorously it seemed implausible that it didn't pop out every time. Suffused with a new frequency of feeling, I sighed. In that dark room, looking down over the dark city, the past and future contracted around the present and this new sovereign fact of my life and the world: there was a person where there hadn't been one before.

This book is about something very ordinary. The facts of the conception, gestation, birth, and neonatal care of my two daughters, beyond a few factors (donor, IVF) were not so unusual. Every person has participated in gestation in one or both roles; we've all *been* gestated at the very least. These matters are commonplace. These ideas have been offered and received, traded freely among those who need them. For all that, they remain surprisingly unwritten. This absence of record is structural: thousands of generations of postpartum thoughts have been whispered out into the night sky while their thinkers sit cradling newborns or pace the floor, hands at nine and six occupied with gentle bouncing, unable to reach for pen and paper. I have written these words mostly between the hours of four and seven a.m., an ear on each child. The work's soundscape has been the almost inaudible push and pull of unobstructed infant breathing. I've periodically stepped away from the page to help a small still-tired body fall back asleep, pressing myself to hold onto my thoughts as I rock or nurse.

The urgency has come from my sense that this book had to be the work of the postpartum period. The writing work is part of the bodywork particular to this time, marked by its knifing pains and disorienting joys, the magnitude of feeling, now overwhelming fear, now befuddling adoration, structured by this period's particular cadence of interruptions. It had to be now because my experience with my first child taught me that these thoughts don't stay. They evaporate as pregnancy and neonatal care recede. For you, for us, I wanted to write this before the things that I want most to record here get sealed in time, folded into my own little underground psychic history. Pregnancy, labor, and delivery become a story that you tell yourself again and again. In the tellings, naturally, the experiences themselves change. I want to engage with those months and days before my stories quite swallow what happened.

I had to write about what it is like. You assume such a record must exist, but I couldn't find one that resonated with me. In part because of the very structural conditions of neonatal care, though the gestating body is obliquely discussed endlessly, any direct engagement with its realities are lost in the harsh light of hyperfocus on superficial emblems: celebrity baby bumps and the bang of gender reveal parties. The pregnant body is hypervisible and the individual pregnant person feels themself the object of so much looking. But this constant attention has not served to generalize knowledge about this bodily habit that has inducted so many into such a diversity of identities and rituals. *What is this thing that gestates?* The material investigations that would provide answers are displaced by ethical and political matters that are not essential to the experience but are rather hung on gestation. Media depictions and politicians' talking points laden gestation with meanings that stand instead of observations made most often by those most involved. The history of philosophy is rife with metaphors of conception, gestation, and birth. But, these metaphors don't grow out of the experiences themselves. An account of what this *is* has been displaced by endless claims about what this *means* in collective understanding.

So, in this book, I try to excavate what this experience is from the vast accumulation of what it is said to mean. This explanation does not stem from a medical account; the empiricism here isn't in the way medical language explains what is happening in our bodies, although the process involves learning in this regard. Rather the empiricism is experiential. The thought stems from sensation, observation, and most importantly from conversation, from how these experiences were clarified by the guidance of others who'd had these and related experiences. I set out to understand — through writing — conception, gestation, birth, and postpartum as processes against the static image of the mother and what she is made to represent rhetorically and politically. I narrate gestation as an unfolding against the consequential terms in which pregnancy has been deemed a state of being. So, in sum: this book names what an unfolding process is against an almost exclusive cultural focus on what a static state of being means. You might say that this book seeks to rescue gestation from pregnancy.

What are these forces that have made this often-looked-at thing so difficult to see clearly? Essay One, "Fetal Separateness," suggests that one significant factor is the conversion of this human experience into an issue for judgments, policies, and regulations. The essay works back from the logic and claims of the Supreme Court decision, concurrences, and dissents in *Dobbs v. Jackson Women's Health* to uncover the genealogy of this conversion of intimate bodily matters into state concerns. The essay is entitled "Fetal Separateness" because, from *Roe* and *Casey* — decisions that were celebrated for guaranteeing and maintaining the legality of abortion — the question of when a fetus could be feasibly extracted from the body of a gestator has been a central concern in regulating, and thereby legitimizing, the right to abortion. The essay contrasts the interpretations of personhood and autonomy that were so central to the jurisprudential approach to abortion (and therefore the premises of the politics of abortion) with the provocations on these topics that gestation itself produces.

To see the reality of gestating bodies freed of their overdetermined cultural inscription is to see that bodies are biological entities defined by constant change. Under the layers of mystification and naturalization that attend feminizing processes dwell bodies that are not somehow abruptly categorically different from other bodies upon conception. Rather, pregnancy modifies the body in a way that must be recognized in its reality: as sex modification, both endocrinological and morphological. Adjusting organic chemical flows, reconfiguring organs, opening or sealing shut tubes for a desired effect: these processes connect gestation to other forms of bodily change. Essay Two, "Is a Cervix Cis?" suggests that this process of body modification, *contra* the long history of viewing uteruses and breasts as trans-historical sources of pain and degradation, provides a way out of the strictures of assigned sex, opening up language that provides a more accurate account of the experience of embodiment. Right in this state in which the body has been the most mystified, there are resources that contradict both the containment of the gestating body in the misogynist scripts that history has written and the cordoning off of bodies into two essential and opposite types.

This liberatory implication of gestation extends to the distinct work of neonatal care, which, like uteruses and breasts, has often been presented as a snare of unfreedom. Essay Three, "The Hydraulics of Provision," finds in the activity of breastfeeding a theory regarding the social forms through which needs, and even wants, can be met absent the paradigm of labor. The hydraulic process of nursing models a social hydraulics where demand determines supply and routinely recalibrates to avoid surplus. Both terms in this system, the baby and the person who lactates, participate in this work, and the wellness of each is necessary to its successful execution. The incursion of work on the scene of neonatal care interrupts this balance and throws both the lactator and the child into physical and emotional distress. The thrumming hum of the breast pump in the office or workplace bathroom is the best-case scenario, more often early cessation is necessary. The essay proposes that all of life could be engaged with the acts of provision, a form which, against common depictions, does away with the distinction between the provider and the provided for.

This book, which is about the provocations produced through careful engagement with the material experience of gestating new life, ends with death. The fourth and final essay, "Wars, Wars, Wars; or Swimming in the Waters of the World," works back through the wars waged on the people of the world by the American government during my early years of life.[1] Dragging this backdrop of the everyday to the fore reveals the context for every act of provision or care in the world as it is currently organized. Our deathcult of war, our easy material support for genocides and dictators, is simply the opposite of gestation. This is the material work of sorting out who is yours (and you are therefore bound to protect) and who is not yours (and therefore among those who you must protect your own against). This essay concludes with the simple observation that the first encounter with a neonate following birth or the first meeting with a child who will come into your care is an encounter with a stranger. A miracle of gestation and birth is that you can love a stranger. The gestational sensorium — the feeling and gestures proper to the work of keeping a child alive and well, both *in utero* and *in mundo* — offers a total antagonism against the endless, child-killing state of war.

* * *

I was shocked by the wateriness of the whole thing. "To my knowledge, all humans in history have been manufactured underwater," writes Sophie Lewis in "Amniotechnics," the text I read in the postpartum ward as my six-hour-old daughter lay in her cotton swaddle next to me.[2] The manufacture is just the beginning. There was the iconic instance; the first trickle of amniotic fluid fell onto my feet and the sidewalk as we waited for the cab to the hospital ("Is it raining?" I asked my partner, putting out my hand). A full rush of an emptied uterus followed on the delivery bed, a reality as self-evident as a river. Despite the centrality of water-breaking to the cultural script of birth, both times that it happened to me, I was surprised.

There's the sweat from the hours of effort. The wetness of the baby as she's put on your chest, her skin and visage soft, mouth opening and shutting, used to getting what she needs from water. The smell of delivery is something like the herpetarium house at the zoo, the odor of creatures biologically destined to be terrestrial but still sliding around in water, skin infused with their aqueous environment. There's the postpartum dampness. For the day or two following an uncomplicated vaginal delivery, you lie in the hospital bed with a steady flow of fluid soaking thick absorbent pads manufactured for this purpose. An event of the first day is your attention to your body as you undress for your first shower, the water so welcome and also painful. Providers come and push on your deflating abdomen to encourage rushes of fluid. This fluid, which is called lochia, weeps out of your body for weeks in progressively paler hues: first bright red (lochia rubra), then pink (lochia serosa), and finally white (lochia alba). You follow the progression of this watery ombre to confirm that you are healing internally. This is the beginning of the wateriness of the subsequent years: breastmilk, spit up, throw up, pee, liquid poop, snot, drool, food that becomes gradually less liquid everywhere. A halo of sweat around the head tells you that your sleeping child is too warm.

Then there was the vast well of tears, the material manifestation of the wateriness of feeling. My first daughter and I had difficulty nursing. As a result, she had difficulty maintaining weight in those first days. In the days following her birth, every time I thought of her weight I would be so overcome with fear that first I would go limp, unable to speak, then my mouth would set to trembling. Then the well would open, and

I would be sobbing freely. Even now, writing these words, I'm transported to the terror and anguish of seeing an ounce decrease on the doctor's scale, all our hours of work together unable to keep pace with the demand of the hours for calories.

The second baby, lusciously fat, easy with nursing, gaining impressively, found me likewise crying freely, but with none of the force of the sobbing, just a steady leaking out of my eyes. I was even able to converse normally through the flood, talking and laughing as I wiped away the salty water. The volume again expressed my degree of feeling, now of a different kind. It was relief this time; my body was saying *I can't believe that this one is thriving. Can you believe it?*

The wateriness expressed something else that was new in me: that I would never be happy again. Never happy again because even though my baby was well, and I rejoiced in this, I still knew that not every baby through all of time was or had been. How to express that it wasn't just my babies that I cried for in terror and delight, reader, it was also for the baby that you were? Maybe your caregiver carried you, your hair covered in the cement dust from a building crushed by American-funded bombs. Maybe you were taken from your family by a state bureaucracy whose policy is to kidnap children from their families and communities. Maybe you were sick and neglected; surely you were sometimes hungry, scared, or cold. And what of the millions and millions of babies who have died in their vulnerability?

Newly, such facts of history became the only facts of history. Like the historian emerita who deals in ages named for their corresponding English monarchs, I wanted to reorder the past to monumentalize the names of dead children. Fie the Elizabethan Age, that was the time when Jane Blackman died of plague. They weren't the Obama years, that was the epoch of Trayvon Martin. How can so pure a tragedy as any single child's death remain unattended by collective mourning and

PREFACE: US

unproductive of collective purpose? How is it that every such death does not substantially change history? Now, it seemed to me, the only way to trace what had been, was, or would be was through the unending scroll of names of children the world had harmed.

It was thus that the world itself became newly intolerable to me. From a person ruled by rational thought, I became the infrastructure of a biologically induced militancy. I was newly radicalized, re-radicalized, brought into an absolute antagonism with what humankind has wrought by, so it seemed, my glands and the chemical feedback between myself and the delicate creatures who I felt the compulsion to tent with my own sturdy, established body. The child was not the emblem, but the occasion, the provocateur, the teaser out of the chemicals that did this to me. It was she, and later, they two whose enchanting existence disenchanted me. It was their very singularity, each of them, that provided scale for the general loss, the infinite magnitude of lost singularities.

This contraction of the general and the particular is common; I see others experience it. I can't hold my babies, talk to them, or assess their needs without feeling the interchangeability of their particular bodies with the bodies of children that the powerful are bent on destroying or letting die. One form this interchangeability takes is the visual hallucinations that come in flashes: the overlay of their faces on those of other babies, or of other baby faces on theirs. The force of this eminently clarifying confusion produces a physical jolt to the heart, a pang. It is a cousin to the reactive gesture to unzip the coat of a baby who I think seems too hot on the subway, the physical impulse to run to catch a new walker who I'm worried will fall as she toddles behind a sibling, the twitch to scoop up a child who slips from the monkey bars. It comes when scrolling through the internet in the middle of the night and seeing (unspeakably, how can I write this?) the limp bodies of dead children, who in their death look so much like they are just sleeping, like they are the child sleeping next to me. It comes in the recurring dreams on those rare nights when REM sleep is achieved, dreams of those loved bodies in pain. It comes in the panic of waking with a scream stuck in my throat and my pulse racing, in the tears cried alone as I touch the heads of my sleeping children, unable to habituate myself to the reality that they are, indeed, alive and safe. Newly, I'm unwilling to allow the reality of their relative safety to soothe me. Cultivating this unwillingness has come to be, for me, the constitutive act of mothering.

You can hone the skill of dissociation, a cruel or a tender dissociation, in order to live and surely there must be some of that. Or, this book suggests, you can also lean closer to your friend at the bar in the odd hour you've scraped together to see them or on the text thread of pictures of healthy round babies playing and say: you're right to feel this way. We are right to feel this way. If anything, we could feel it more. The world of stupid, constant cruelty is the same world that devastates and deprives us and ours. Just as we can't accept mass death, we don't have to settle for the two hours together in between work, when we (exhausted) pick them up (exhausted) from childcare and go home to make dinner, feed them, bathe them, and collapse in bed. Floor dinner, as I call it to the disgust of my co-parent, is my little joke that is not a joke about mostly eating only what's left after my children eat. I shouldn't do this and I shouldn't have to. We don't have to acquiesce to the slow poisoning of our children and ourselves via water and air. We don't have to participate in the racist, anti-poor fantasy, fed to us to distract from these monumental general threats, that we can shore up the safety and wellness of our children by honing indifference to the safety and wellness of other people's children. We can follow our instinct to love as love loves, which is to say hugely with an accelerant force that breaks the world as it is. I've seen in the eyes and heard in the words of my friends the radicalizing effects of caring for young children. This is just one iteration of the way that naming the conditions of the world as it is makes this everyday intolerable. It was through these tired, beautiful friends that I came to know that these changes were not only produced by chemicals. Rather, my impulses and impressions only cohered when my friends mirrored them back to me. Only when my childcare experiences were held in common, held in sympathy, did I understand their true nature.

Even as it washed over me, I felt that postpartum anxiety is a political feeling. It's the refusal to contain your newfound realization that your personhood extends beyond your skin to the individual person who has occasioned this realization. This state is the refusal of the reality that your constant vigilance can't save all of the children, in fact, you can't do anything for most of them. It's the refusal to countenance that the buffalo stampede of human vulnerability is waterfalling over the cliff of social indifference to life itself. You can stand at cliff's edge watching, waving your arms, but you will not stop the flow or be able to catch even one, so needful is every individual human life.

So, this book embedded in me in the bright light of the drugstore aisle. A few days postpartum with my first baby, as my first re-engagement with the commerce of the world, I walked to Rite Aid for diapers, size newborn, for my diminished daughter. Exiting the dim cave of neonatal care, in which night and day were no longer distinct, in which softness of touch, sound, and smell reigned over this indistinction, the six blocks of walking were a lesson in my new sensitivity. The loudness of a motorcycle engine, the smell of summer garbage, the clunking vibrations of the 7 train and the screech of brakes, the brightness of August: all these normal city stimuli, frightening, bewildering, overloading my nervous system many times over. This harshness was enmeshed with my first experience of separation, the stretch of the tether excruciating. *Where was this part of me that wasn't anymore? Where was this new creature, my baby?* If she was not here, she must be alone. She could be dying.

I resisted the consuming urge to run back to her. I had to tell myself that I was an adult with a mind. I needed to keep walking, to get diapers, to keep her dry and clean. I arrived in the baby aisle. Next to the diapers was the shelf of infant formula. The canisters of brand name formula were priced at $34.99 and the drugstore generic $29.99. All the canisters were fitted with anti-theft devices. When I saw these objects that communicated the efforts of the Rite Aid corporation to prevent caretakers who didn't have enough money to buy the formula from stealing the formula, reality broke. In a flash, the suffering implied in this image of a tub of the only substance that could sustain the most vulnerable life locked in a cage unspooled the suffering of every child in the world, their hunger and thirst. This, in turn, unspooled the suffering of every child who has ever suffered.

In the four pandemic years since that day, everyone living in the United States (and this, I've come to realize, is very much a book of and about that country) has become habituated to the general lockdown of drugstore commodities. Most of the items for sale in Rite Aid that heal or keep a body well, clean, or nourished have been placed behind plastic panels. Now you need to press a button to call over one of the few remaining harried employees in the eerily underpopulated robot stores to unlock the panels so that you can buy your pain reliever or your toothbrush. But, infant formula was the canary in the coal mine of deprivation; it was one of the first products to be treated in this way.

So, perhaps primarily, this book is an expression of thirst. Its urgency is an analog to the state you're in when a fussy newborn finally latches, and bracing your body, immobilized lest your nipple again fall out of the tiny mouth, you're struck with a spontaneous dehydration panic, the urgent need to immerse your whole head in a horse trough. You're so thirsty, so unable to move toward water. This book scorns the parching failure of liberalism to imagine any adequate freedom and expresses the fine freedom that gestation, birth, and childcare have offered me personally, prefiguring a finer and more general freedom to come. Of course, my observations are particular, not universal. They arise in the context of my own experiences and my own iteration of a renewed desire for the world's future. But they represent experiences that were plumped with meaning because I found their reflection in the words of other people who had gestated, cared for children, or cared for my children. By this last I mean those who have loved my children, whose lives were, like mine expanded by their arrival.

So, no, not universal but extremely common, often communicated but unrecorded. Gestation is the physical making of a person. The work that we call pregnancy is only a relatively short stage of this project. For some of us, the project of gestation ends at birth. For others, the physical work of making a person begins at birth or at some point after. This book suggests that careful engagement with the continuities between gestation in the uterus and gestation in the world contains oracular wisdom. The long history of mystifying this experience, a fake fixation on it, a false monumentalizing, has prevented the serious engagement that is necessary to unlock its conceptual provocations.

The common thoughts that gestation brings can help us to imagine a room, an apartment, a building, a block, a neighborhood, a city, a world in which we collectively put down the task of producing accumulation for the rich and take up the project of reproducing each other. Perhaps these thoughts can come in even the most unlikely rooms. The shock to the system of loving felt by so many as they begin to care for a child provides a paradigm for social feeling and social structures, and, in the long winter that awaits us, this resource might be worth turning towards. In this area of life that has been most thoroughly annexed by the catastrophically failed project of liberal feminism — formed as it is by the stupefactions of white supremacy, settler colonialism, and capitalist lifeways — we find resources that could reorient those energies toward genuine, general feminist freedom.

I said at the beginning of this preface that the pronoun *us* regained its grammatical coherence following birth and that's true, but it's an incomplete truth. *Us* changed once and in the hours, days, months, and years that followed the miraculous entry of my children into the world, it has changed again. The recontouring of *us* that gestation and birth precipitated has become thrillingly and excruciatingly general. Because, in millions of dark rooms all over the world, at this precise moment, caring for newborns is making inescapable the reality that the priorities and practices dictated by the powerful are incompatible with life at every level. But, it is also an experience that can whisper back into the dark of a caregiver's four a.m.: you are not alone. We are not alone. What we feel for our children can amplify, diffuse, and saturate. The feeling doesn't need to stay at home. The *us* that is reproduced when we care for a child can multiply until it's simply the sole stuff of our collective lives.

— Queens, May 2025

One: Fetal Separateness

> I am afraid to own a Body —
> I am afraid to own a Soul —
> Profound — precarious Property
> — Emily Dickinson, Poem 1090

On December 1, 2021, "persons having business before the honorable, the Supreme Court of the United States" argued their positions in the case of *Dobbs v. Jackson Women's Health*.[1] For two hours that winter morning, I lay on the green couch in my living room, silently listening to the live-stream of those arguments with my four-month-old baby asleep on my chest, thin legs encircling my waist, soft bald head nestled under my chin, her mouth slightly open, lightly snoring. The justices' questions and lawyers' answers focused on things august men have written: laws concerning abortion stretching back to the pre-founding foundations of American law and the personal right to liberty and physical autonomy in that same tradition. The real living baby shifted slightly on my abdomen, interrupting the alternate world of the legal arguments in which the idea of a baby is sometimes evoked and her reality is nowhere to be found. These exchanges muddled my thinking, reordering the real experience of the previous thirteen months into a mystified timeline between two invented moments: quickening and viability. As I listened, my baby was situated only inches from where she had been when in my body four months before. She was only a few pounds heavier. The jerky motion of her limbs were still those that developed *in utero*. She still seemed surprised by the world she woke many times a day to find that she was inhabiting. The closest these arguments came to addressing the whoosh of a heartbeat or the crimson flood of the birthing room were these two words: quickening and viability. Both lawyers and justices were trying to convert them into legal concepts, in a long tradition of performing this conversion. They centered irrelevant histories and parsed irrelevant words. It felt to me like these performances were covering the ancestral secrets of birth: quickening is not a moment, it's a diffuse terrain of feeling. Viability doesn't make sense as a line. Rather, the concept is invented to cover the intricate work of thriving done by the hybrid body of pregnancy and the sustained bodily involvement of the child and the caretaker after birth.

Six months later, the Court decided in favor of *Dobbs* and the state of Mississippi. Six months after that and one year since I sat listening to the arguments pinned down by my baby, I spent December 2022 in my home state of Wisconsin, where, following the Court's decision, an 1849 law against feticide had gone back into effect, halting abortion care in the state while the courts considered what constitutes killing a baby. By this time, I was pregnant again and joined the millions of people who contemplated the real possibility of pregnancy outcomes in which providers would let us bleed out on a gurney or our organs would fail as our body became overtaken by the infection of miscarried tissue or our fallopian tubes are allowed to burst from the pressure of an ectopic pregnancy while state authorities interpreted 175-year-old laws. I felt in common with the millions of other people who were being denied elective abortions and so faced a different kind of fear, a different modality of the state commandeering our bodily wellness and thereby our lives. Again, as the year before, rhetoric and abstractions clashed with sharp bodily sensations. Again, there was an eerie familiarity to these strangers — past and present — daring to involve themselves in bodily concerns of which they seemed so naively ignorant and yet were so visceral to me. Writing and remembering I rub these two Decembers together in my mind. In the first, my first child and I, recently detached and yet supremely connected, sat together as I listened to nine judges and two lawyers adjudicate what we are and who has jurisdiction over our bodies. In the second, my body was once again this modified place taken up by constant discussion that said nothing about the subject at hand. Holding a child without, holding a fetus within: I was the same person, wasn't I?

What is gestation to the gestator? This simple, essential question is largely unanswered in public discussion because it is largely unasked. In its place is the interminable repetition of other questions. As the original origin point, the eternally renewable emblem of all beginnings, philosophers and pundits assign pregnancy the burden of holding the most fundamental religious, philosophical, and ethical truths. In public debate about this activity, we are invited to continually search for the answers to questions that are unanswerable outside of a metaphysical frame: What delimits a human life? What defines a human soul? How is animacy breathed into matter? Or more prosaically: What are the essential values of a particular society? How should moral questions relate to politics in a supposedly secular democracy? In these more earthly registers, the questions take for granted the jurisprudential consensus that gestation is a productive activity in which the state has a vested interest. For the liberal politics of gender, gestation is a vulnerability that exposes gestators to limitations to their worldly advancement and success. Gestation is none of these things in itself, and it is precisely what gestation is in itself that this essay seeks to illuminate.

To pose the answerable questions, to ask simply, What is this process? What are its moods and sensations? What are its aesthetics and socialities? What do gestators do and what does gestation do to them? These questions seem impossible, corny, medical at best but too intimate to take up any space in sober public debate. The process itself, then, is peculiarly situated: both central and unimportant, essential in terms of implications, but in itself unworthy of investigation. It seems that pregnancy is too personal to ground anything as real as policy in the individual material instance. Yet, as an abstraction, it is available for constant public comment. These public claims are, in fact, made most often by those farthest from it in material and experiential terms. Do you know how to assess the state of your cervical mucus and why you would try? If you have ever desired, pursued, or achieved pregnancy you very likely do. Now, imagine Samuel Alito, associate justice of the U.S. Supreme Court and author of the majority opinion that ended the constitutional protection for abortion, saying the phrase "cervical mucus."

The materiality of gestation is not wholly absent from the landscape of public attention; there are two primary forms in which descriptions of fetuses and gestation are common; both focus on abortion. First, the fetus is central to the political culture of social conservatives. On a rural highway near where I grew up in central Wisconsin, an uncaptioned billboard contrasts a pink fetus with a red background lit from behind, implying the availability of much more detailed and colorful imaging of the uterine environment than one gets from ultrasound. On another billboard, visible from the bike route of my commute through Queens, a caption alongside a photograph of a headless pregnant abdomen informs viewers that real men choose life.

Anti-abortion tables have been a familiar site on every college campus where I've worked, nestled among those of Greek organizations and other clubs. They display photographs of aborted fetal tissue blown up and affixed to posts like liturgical banners. Plastic models representing the stages of fetal development are arranged on a table, inviting care for the live beings with translucent pink skin. Such galleries often line major thoroughfares through campus, necessitating that students and staff walk the gauntlet to get to classrooms and offices. The social conservative political movement, since it discovered abortion as an issue that could unite its factions in the late 1970s, has centered the fetus as the protagonist of pregnancy. In this frame, the politics of pregnancy begin and end with the enforcement of the imperative to remain pregnant regardless of inclination or capacity. The health of any individual person's pregnancy and the sum total of what comes after — the wellness of young parents, infants, and children — be damned.

The right wing has also claimed the emotional landscape of gestation. The movement is largely concerned with public displays of pathos, with the imperiled fetus again at the center of its care. This essay aims to relocate the deeply resonant emotional aspects of gestation, birth, and neonatal care in those experiences themselves, rather than in the sentimentalizing interpretations of those engaged in one of the most enduringly successful bait-and-switch schemes in recent politics: aggrandizing gestation and mothering in their rhetoric while materially abandoning both mothers and the children to a steadily escalating austerity.

Pope John Paul II popularized the phrase "the culture of life" in two encyclicals written in 1991 and 1995 to galvanize Catholic self-concept and purpose. This phrase drew together anti-choice politics with the promotion of marriage and opposition to the death penalty. There is, perhaps, no purer commandeering of the ethical as such than the suggestion that one's politics are for life. And yet, it's not the scope but rather the content of the claim that is objectionable. I aim to provide another vocabulary for engaging with the material reality of gestation as a question of life, for knowing the fetus and the gestator. The physical elements of pregnancy — fetal tissue and uterine environments — are not a problem for a politics of choice to overcome. Rather, many of us experience a greater understanding and commitment to ensuring abortion access during and following pregnancy. Intimacy with the provocations around life and personhood that pregnancy provokes are, in fact, the ground for a politics of life that are very different from those suggested by the Pope and his ideological brethren.

Lately, there has been a revival of a second primary political context for the circulation of unabstracted images and descriptions of gestation. Since the June 2022 ruling in *Dobbs*, to consume American media in any medium or ideological register is to consume descriptions of pregnancy-related difficulties that have been allowed to progress to emergencies due to either restriction on abortion care or confusion about the rules that govern the provision of abortion care in a particular state. How many times have we wept silently, sitting in our cars or on the subway, as we listened to women recount in the most graphic physical detail, often not for the first or last time, an experience that combined perhaps the most profound emotional anguish of their lives with severe physical pain and fear of their own death? Surely we all have a mental file of images generated by post-*Dobbs* pregnancy horror stories. I have been collecting a folder of such stories on my computer.

We have been obliged to imagine ourselves in the position of Brittany Watts, to select one of many examples. In September 2023, Watts arrived in an emergency room following the rupture of her membranes at twenty-one weeks gestation with a high white blood cell count. She was made to wait on a gurney for eight hours while blood and amniotic fluid leaked out of her vagina, returning home in this state of agonizing confusion, only to return the next day to spend eleven hours on a gurney while a medical ethics board determined whether a doctor should be allowed to remove the non-viable fetus from her uterus. They ultimately decided that they would not do so before a physician determined that she was "at high risk of bleeding and or serious infection that could lead to death."[2] She returned home to miscarry that fetal tissue into a toilet, which she then scooped into a bucket, and in the emotional and physical state of someone who has been bleeding for two days, attempted to clean the blood off the floor of her bathroom, alone. She returned to the emergency room to seek care, only to have the nurse who had been rubbing her back to comfort her call the police. They would search her home, find the fetal remains in her toilet, arrest her and charge her with desecration of a corpse. It is one thing to be horrified by these stories. It is another to be able to feel the physical pain that Brittany Watts must have felt, the extreme cramping and nausea. Consider the physical vulnerability and the indignity of being observed and discussed for two days, over the course of many hours through the very personal and physical process of miscarrying.

It's only in these horror stories that the fetus — as fetus — is allowed its reality. Advocating for the right to abortion has long taken the form of the most ghastly physical descriptions. The choice of the coat hanger as a political symbol going back to the 1960s is part of this tradition. We all have holes at the center of our bodily infrastructure. For a moment, imagine inserting the unfurled end of a metal hanger into your body just there and rooting around until blood starts to run free. The recent political situation requires a revival of this imaginative tradition.

From the moment that abortion entered federal law, conservative and liberal jurists agree that the state has an interest in pregnancy. The camps disagree about when this interest begins. For conservatives, when egg and sperm meet, before implantation, a baby exists. This person is entitled to all the rights and protections of any other person. For this milieu, pregnancy in itself is not a politics but is the occasion for politics, a vessel for oblique reference to matters primarily of race, money, and the maintenance of an intergenerationally reproduced power structure. The doctrine of fetal personhood has attempted to create legal interpretations and social structures that extend rights and protections so that they come into effect at the moment of fertilization.[3] It is the pregnant person who is the primary risk to these rights and protections. The fetus then, is an antagonist to the gestator, to the extent that there is a gestator, to the extent that she is not yet simply a mother.

In the liberal legal formulation, gestation is the process between fertilization and the moment that a fetus could be wrested from the body of the gestator and conceivably survive. After this moment, the fetus can be viewed as an individual and therefore states have the right to regulate abortions after this point. Until recently, there has been wide concession to the sovereign importance of viability, that fantasized moment when the fetus could be conceivably removed from the gestating uterus and thrive. Seven states at the time of writing do not have limits on post-viability abortions; the recognition that such limits are acceptable and reasonable is central to the *Dobbs* dissent.

Rather than an enormously consequential social process that ought to be understood and supported, for conservatives, pregnancy is an activity of state interest and so subject to state control. For mainstream pro-choice messengers, the politics of pregnancy primarily comes down to the right not to be pregnant. Beginning with the Clinton administration's concessions to social conservatives in his signature accomplishment of welfare reform, for both groups, beyond abortion, pregnancy enters politics when individual women do it too many times with too few resources. Pregnancy *qua* pregnancy seems not apolitical but antipolitical.

There are also conservative and liberal iterations of the claim that biology gives a transhistorical character to the labors of childbirth and childcare that has long limited women's freedom. These tendencies agree that gestation is a private affair. For conservatives, this limitation is correct and empirical; it ought, therefore, to structure society into male wage earners and female homemakers. For liberals, who have oriented their legal and political arguments around privacy, this delimitation is an unfortunate tradition that disadvantages women and ought to be transcended. To these liberals, to the extent that gestation enters politics, it does so as a risk factor. This capacity makes a person vulnerable to decreased earning potential or containment in the domestic sphere. Political reform means providing her with the means to leave her gestationality at home and venture into the world of public values unhampered by all those soft feelings and incalculable labors that don't belong there.

But let us retreat from these limited terms in which we've been invited to view gestation and begin again: *What is gestation to the gestator? What is a fetus if it is not a person, but cannot be adequately or exhaustively described as just tissue?* Gestation is a story, but whose, and of what kind? This experience is first an act of the gestator's narrative imagination. When it begins in the little-known territory of your own uterus, the story might take the form of a plaint: *this can't be happening; please let this stop happening.* Or it might be a plea: *please, don't stop happening; I want very much for this to keep happening.* You might hope that you can ignore this abstraction and it will go away. You might hold the idea of this microscopic entity in your mind all day like a delicate ember, visualizing the interior of the organ it inhabits, believing that your sheer will can gently oxygenate it into ignition and lasting vigor. You might move through your days with the worry that hitting a pothole on your bike will dislodge this abstraction or accidentally taking a bite of soft cheese will poison it. All the while, you envision the invisible zygote embedding itself into the wall of tissue that is the only real first-hand experience with the material reality of what's happening inside your body. You've been attuned to that tissue leaking or surging out of your body for years. Perhaps, for years, in a pinch, you've ducked around a corner to put your hand down your pants and come out with a hand covered in blood.

For a long time, the process only shows itself in sensations that are familiar, but reconfigured, intensified, and prolonged. While you've felt tired before, the first months of gestation often bring a fatigue so profound that you don't get up when the bus reaches your stop because you feel that you can't. If you work in an office, you might lie down on the floor of that office (only to spring up, revolted, when a cockroach the size of a small mouse scurries out from under the radiator toward your head). When you do the grocery shopping you might lean heavily on the cart and consider lying down in the bright light of the supermarket aisle. On the weekend, you might fall asleep at five p.m. and sleep through, if you are able. If you have other care responsibilities or are otherwise unable to rest when you need to rest, the fatigue multiplies and compounds. This new kind of tiredness is the means through which gestation progresses from a fact that you know about your body to an experience that you're having in your body.

Then, there's the reordering of your senses. For six, eight, twelve, sixteen weeks or more, you might feel as you do when you have the stomach flu, except that when you throw up you don't experience the familiar window of relief. It had been six years since I'd thrown up when I arrived at my first pregnancy. I remember because the time previous was the morning after drinking too much whiskey following the memorial of a beautiful friend who died in a jail cell tragically, early, and in great physical and emotional pain.

You wake up in the morning with sour nausea as your first conscious perception. Your trigger foods become your enemies. Common triggers include cheese, eggs, meat, vegetables, coffee, and milk. For me almost every edible or drinkable substance was a trigger. You must force yourself to eat the few things that remain palatable because an empty stomach intensifies the sickness. Awake in the night, sitting on the lip of the bathtub head in hands, saltine cracker crumbs flecking your nightgown, you try wild-eyed and in vain to stay ahead of it. You might try to nap to escape it or, unable to sleep, just sink into the misery all day long.

The smell of the perfume of a stranger with whom you wait to cross the street or a note of someone's sandwich that you're newly able to detect from across a large room devastates your olfactory system. You sprint the hallways to throw up in the office bathroom. You try to be discreet while throwing up in the bushes as you walk to the train. You throw up in a plastic juice pitcher that your clever and experienced mother gave you so that you could vomit safely while stuck in traffic when that became necessary. With my second pregnancy, I was often caring for my toddler during this period. Several times, I set her up with a toy in the hall as I knelt over the toilet, saying "It's okay baby, don't worry" in between bouts. She would inch closer to me, finally sitting on the threshold between the bathroom and the hall six inches from where I knelt. First worried, then curious, eventually, she'd become frustrated by my inattention and begin to cry.

Pregnant people are also unusually vulnerable to gastrointestinal viruses and food-borne pathogens due to the immune suppression that protects the fetus from attack by the pregnant person's body. I had bouts of one or the other of these with both pregnancies. I believe the culprit in the first pregnancy was a pastry purchased from a bakery in the neighborhood where I live and the second was cherries that I purchased from a deli near work. While in the twenty-four hours of throwing up at volume, I remembered how different this kind of nausea is from morning sickness. It is a process of escalating nausea, vomiting, relief, and recovery. Also, because I was deemed *really* sick I was given leave to lie in bed and support with other tasks. I realized how different gastroenteritis is from the interminable experience of morning sickness. Or, many people are spared both, feeling nothing at all for the first months, so I understand. And all this time, what's happening to your body is invisible to the outside world and untellable to all but the few people who you won't mind having known if what is happening all becomes nothing in a sudden bloody rush.

Eventually, for most people, the nausea and vomiting wanes, if unevenly. On a Tuesday afternoon, you might say to yourself with excitement *I only feel a little bit nauseous!* or catch yourself feeling normal for hours at a time, only to wake the next morning defeated by the familiar dread. And for some, it doesn't end. For those who endure *hyperemesis gravidarum* extreme nausea and vomiting lasts until giving birth, often prematurely, or as is the case at the elevated rate of more than a third of these cases, until a pregnancy loss. There is no medical term for this common experience, only for this extreme expression.

This often daily, all-day, consuming experience is colloquially called morning sickness. The absence of its true nature and scale from public consciousness and popular representation becomes very meaningful when you experience it yourself. How can it be that so many people have been walking around in this state all along? How many times was your elementary school teacher stricken by this debilitating fatigue? How many times was your deodorant smell devastating the person who stood beside you in an elevator, unbeknownst to you? There is no socialized accommodation to help the new gestator manage these conditions. There is no public monument to its quotidian endurance. There is no ritual of celebration marking its diminution and cessation. And yet, it is a human experience that has accompanied, to some degree, the passage into the world of 70–80% of human beings.

This phase — the first trimester — is deeply private, in part because it is both (for most) so physically consuming and (for many) largely invisible and secret or, at least, not widely discussed. You have perhaps never been so aware of the fact that your body is a thing. You have perhaps never been so in tune with the way that chemicals produce effects in that body. In these weeks, your body is so insistent, ever present to your notice. It is conspicuous not for the reasons that your body has been previously of notice or will soon be of notice in a newly intense and invasive way: because people look at you and have a reaction or opinion. For once, in pregnancy, you have a bodily experience that is about what your body is, rather than what people think about it. Your body asserts itself to you in particular, often following a life of mostly encountering this thing via the perceptions of others.

Early pregnancy is like athletics in this way. The feeling was similar to me. Like sport, gestation allows you to recognize your body's capacities and changeable nature in a way that, ideally, you seek out and can manage yourself to some degree. Sport is, for many, the only domain in which the body becomes an instrument through which you act rather than a fact to which you must reconcile yourself. You can choose to go harder or easier and use techniques of distraction to manage discomfort. Management of breath is key at several significant points. The process interestingly crystallizes the relation between the physical and the psychological. Its athleticism appears to me also in its extremity, its sometimes uncomfortable intensity, and its emotional lability. It is something you can train for, but mostly only as it's happening. Gestation is, in part, teaching yourself to gestate, submitting to the demands of any particular pregnancy. It seems like a contradiction that pregnancy is also like disability and or rather, perhaps, just is a disability. Its extremes require you to re-evaluate the kinds of ability that structure the built environment and social customs of our everyday.

If you want the pregnancy, and I only ever wanted both of mine, wanted them desperately, actually, then your desire for the process to go forward is probably the primary concern, overriding the difficulties. You can try to foster the process according to medical advice: take walks, sleep as much as possible, hydrate, eat as much and as well as you can, take your prenatal vitamins, limit or eliminate caffeine, strengthen your back, avoid twisting your midsection. You might feel very frustrated by the difficulties and discomforts. For many, I think, it feels like your body is being overtaken. But for me, it felt like something my body was doing with my collaboration and protection. I was grateful to my body for what it was doing. Crucially, this phase is yours to experience and interpret.

Then, after several months of your body's assertions, its insistent presence, you think you feel a meaningful flutter, a pinch, a jab. You pause to try to focus on it. You put your hand on the place where you think you felt something, but are probably still unsure, especially if it's your first time. The feeling is subtle at first and almost indistinguishable from other feelings: turnings of the stomach and intestines, pains of your expanding uterus, and the pinches of stretching abdominal muscles. To understand if what you're feeling is fetal movement, you consult others who have gestated.

It might take several weeks, but these movements disarticulate from the other bodily feelings. Gradually, you become certain that you are feeling something new. These sensations become distinguishable, singular. First they are gentle. Then, day by day, week by week they become stronger. If you want the pregnancy to continue you might start clocking your life in these fluttering jabs, the frequency and strength of which, according to your doctor's advice, indicate the health of the fetus. How many per hour? Are they enough? Do they feel vigorous? If you catch yourself realizing that you haven't felt movement in a while, you may get worried. You have a glass of orange juice, hoping that, per medical advice, the spike in blood sugar will provoke fetal movement. Following the protocol, you quiet your body so you can detect the smallest movements. You lie in the quiet dark waiting, attuned to the feeling of the inside of your abdomen. You might beg. It is during this period that you might stop with a generalized plea for the continuance of the pregnancy and begin to address a specific abstraction: *please keep moving*. It is there in the dark, in the indeterminacy of what is and what may be that you may begin to hope that a person will slowly and by degrees arrive. This is the process through which, from the indistinction between your body and the fetus's body, you begin to recognize a distinction.

A little clump of cells on the screen has become a recognizable profile. You sit in the dark of the imaging wing of the hospital while a sonographer catalogs a list of measurements of organs and limbs, of the space between this and that physiological feature, the proportions of which will indicate something about the development of the fetus. Eventually, you get to know the movement of the fetus around the uterus. Quick jabs of limbs become the swirls of the fetal body turning in the amniotic fluid. In your doctor's office, on the ultrasound screen, you can see a butt, a foot, or a head pushing on this or that quadrant of your belly and feel the corresponding place on your abdomen. "Yep, that's a butt," your obstetrician says as she passes the gel-covered wand over the upper left quadrant and you may see the round shape of a head poking out, "and that is a head," in the lower right. You look at the abstracted figure on the screen, the fetal silhouette and choreography so familiar due to their cultural ubiquity. You look down at your belly distended in this or that quadrant by the fetus's position, perhaps rippling with the movement that you also see on the screen. Sensation syncs with visual impression, a rare instance of experiencing the inside of your body with two senses at once.

You may feel that the fetus is more conceptually available to you than your own gestating body. By this, I mean that this entity in your uterus, the fetus, comes to take on a centrality for you, the gestator, that can eclipse your focus on your own body. When you perform the recommended acts, for example, it is, you imagine, for *them* that you perform these acts. Rather than being able to conceptualize the truth of your body: that it is the site of a process between being one and two, you imagine the fetus as already a separate subject of your care and protection. "Don't worry," the obstetrician told me when I expressed concern that my inability to eat and regular vomiting would nutritionally deprive the embryo and endanger the pregnancy, "she will take everything she needs from you. She will leach the calcium from your bones. If anything you should worry about your body being depleted." I was, in fact, comforted by this information.

Upon further reflection, it is not just the bodies of gestators that disappear from view in public discussion. Perhaps the fetus is not as available as our sense of familiarity with it might suggest. In the influential, vapid political imaginings that have guided so much of what we come to our projects of gestation thinking that we know, the fetus is only available as that which it is not, a baby, or, in the conceptualizing of the right, a fetal person. Another account that reflects the particular effect of the fetus, as a fetus, on the gestator is required. The experience of having a fetus in your body is singular, strange, and instructive. A frank account of that experience is, I suggest, a necessity for a fulsome argument for reproductive justice.

When I'm holding my sleeping children, I often remember a moment during the pregnancy that produced them. My first baby got the hiccups a lot *in utero*. I felt them as a minute rhythmic pulse and once saw them on the sonogram screen. In the days before birth, I dropped a box and I felt her start in my uterus, a sudden jerk. My second baby was consistently active. Her movements felt like gymnastics. Adrienne Rich's description sparks recognition in me. In pregnancy, she writes that she did not:

> experience the embryo as decisively internal ... but rather, as something inside and of me, yet becoming hourly and daily more separate, on its way to becoming separate from me and of itself. In early pregnancy the stirring of the fetus felt like ghostly tremors of my own body, later like the movements of a being imprisoned in me; but both sensations were my sensations, contributing to my own sense of physical and psychic space.[4]

Rich's account calls out for conceptual engagement; if bodies can experience this development of movement, how should we understand that process? What does this experience contribute to understanding the fetus at the intersection of the available concepts: a living part of a person, tissue that can be shed or removed, or an individual person?

The text of the American Supreme Court decisions regarding abortion do not take this question and other questions derived from pregnancy as their objects for adjudication. It is these decisions that contain the framing for public discussion of the politics of pregnancy. The legal history of approaching this process from 1973 to 2022, from *Roe* until *Dobbs*, focused on the "point of viability" as a dividing line. This line was established by Justice Blackmun in his majority opinion in *Roe* after his own and his clerks' non-expert investigations into pregnancy at the Mayo Clinic, and despite the absence of a focus on viability in the lawyers' arguments in the case. The search for a reasonable line after which abortion could be limited came from the centrality of "quickening" to pre-twentieth-century legal frameworks. Justice Blackmun writes for the majority that: "it is undisputed that, at common law, abortion performed before 'quickening' — the first recognizable movement of the fetus *in utero*, appearing usually from the 16th to the 18th week of pregnancy — was not an indictable offense."[5] The legal tolerance of pre-quickening abortion reflected "a confluence of earlier philosophical, theological, and civil and canon law concepts of when life begins."[6] In these areas of thought life's starting point was at some point between conception and live birth when the "embryo or fetus became 'formed' or recognizably human," or in terms of when a "person" came into being, that is, infused with a "soul" or "animated."[7] Until the nineteenth century, Christian theology and canon law "[fixed] the point of animation at forty days for a male and eighty days for a female."[8] This legal framework depended on the idea that, before quickening, "the fetus was to be regarded as part of the mother, and its destruction, therefore, was not homicide" and this basic frame became received common law in the United States.[9]

On this basis, Blackmun's *Roe* opinion developed the viability standard. It was at the point of viability that "the State's important and legitimate interest in potential life" becomes "compelling" because it is following viability that "the fetus then presumably has the capability of meaningful life outside the mother's womb" and therefore "state regulation protective of fetal life after viability thus has both logical and biological justifications" and individual states may therefore "proscribe abortion during that period, except when it is necessary to preserve the life or health of the mother."[10] The notion of viability guided the construction of the trimester framework under which states could not regulate abortion during the first trimester, could do so in the second trimester if doing so in service of the well-being of the pregnant person, and could regulate or outlaw abortion in the third trimester unless the abortion was necessary for the health or life of the pregnant person.

The 1992 opinion in *Planned Parenthood v. Casey* affirmed the central holdings of *Roe* while elevating the concept of viability by doing away with the trimester framework, in part because the decision claimed that changes in medical knowledge would gradually affect at what week of development a fetus could be considered viable. The decision credits the viability line "as a practical matter" with "an element of fairness," and central to this fairness is the consensus that "a woman who fails to act before viability has consented to the State's intervention on behalf of the developing child."[11] The opinion allows states to ban abortion after viability, and to regulate abortion care pre-viability so long as the regulation does not place an undue burden on a pregnant person's ability to decide to have an abortion. The ruling articulates this as allowing states to "enact rules and regulations designed to encourage her to know that there are philosophic and social arguments of great weight that can be brought to bear in favor of continuing the pregnancy to full term and that there are procedures and institutions to allow adoption of unwanted children as well as a certain degree of state assistance if the mother chooses to raise the child herself."[12] In practical terms, from *Casey* until *Dobbs*, conservative states have sought novel ways to limit access to abortion care under the guise of regulating medicine and protecting pregnant women, to avoid court intervention under the undue burden standard.

Then came *Dobbs*. The fundamental argument of Samuel Alito's majority opinion is that there is no American legal tradition of protecting abortion rights. In fact, he contends, *contra Roe* and *Casey* "during ... the period surrounding the enactment of the Fourteenth Amendment — the quickening distinction was abandoned as states criminalized abortion at all stages of pregnancy."[13] Alito's claim is simply counter-factual, according to the most influential history of abortion in the United States, Leslie J. Reagan's *When Abortion Was a Crime*, which is cited in the dissent in *Dobbs*, written by Sonia Sotomayor and signed by Elena Kagan and Stephen Breyer.[14] Pre-quickening abortion criminalization largely targeted purveyors of abortifacients that harmed or killed the gestator and the ethics of the question were largely animated by concern for the gestator.

This dissent also re-emphasized *Casey*'s framing of abortion in terms of women's autonomy. *Casey*, Sotomayor writes:

> recognized the need to extend the constitutional sphere of liberty to a previously excluded group. ... equal citizenship, *Casey* realized, was inescapably connected to reproductive rights. "The ability of women to participate equally" in the "life of the Nation" — in all its economic, social, political, and legal aspects — "has been facilitated by their ability to control their reproductive lives." Without the ability to decide whether and when to have children, women could not — in the way men took for granted — determine how they would live their lives, and how they would contribute to the society around them.[15]

In this strong repudiation of the Alito decision both on the grounds of legal precedent and the grounds of constitutional rights, Sotomayor writes that "coerced pregnancy and birth always impose" a limit on freedom.[16] This limit is measured by the "[diminishing] of women's opportunities to participate fully and equally in the Nation's political, social, and economic life." Sotomayor cites an Amicus Brief by Economists which "show[s] that abortion availability" has "large effects on women's education, labor force participation, occupations, and earnings," as well as "many women's identity and their place in the Nation."[17] The ability to choose abortion "reflects that she is an autonomous person, and that society and the law recognize her as such. ... Beyond any individual choice about residence, or education, or career, her whole life reflects the control and authority that the right grants."[18] I'm very glad that Sotomayer chose to make broad claims in her dissent based on the real effects of abortion access on the material conditions of the lives of people who can become pregnant. My concern is that abortion politics not begin and end in terms dictated by medieval legal precedent and the jurists' hazy understanding of medical realities.

In her book, Reagan argues that the evolution from centering quickening to centering viability tracks with the historical emergence of abortion as a political issue in the late nineteenth century. This politicization was driven by professional organizations of doctors, and specifically obstetricians, who wished to shore up their professional supremacy over homeopaths and midwives in the late nineteenth century as the medical specialty of obstetrics and gynecology was establishing itself with a legitimacy compromised by its association with women's health. The movement characterized non-physician providers as abortionists, which undermined their authority, and this accusation served to distinguish them from quacks and in so doing bolstered their authority as university-trained doctors. Quickening, by definition, is a phenomenon reported by the pregnant person, whereas viability is a line determined by doctors, if roughly.

Reagan describes a concordant shift in understanding of the nature of abortion care. Whereas for centuries women and healthcare providers had regarded menstruation and early pregnancy as contiguous processes, commonly referring to abortion as a process of "restoring the menses," increasingly the termination of pregnancy was described as killing a separate entity. This was the conceptual shift that began to legitimate limits on the procuring and provision of abortion. This development represents the wresting of control over matters of pregnancy and birth from women who possessed inherited knowledge by coalitions of professional men.

The *Dobbs* decision has ushered in a profound acceleration in the scope of this coercion. At the time of writing, twelve states have total bans and seven more have bans before eighteen weeks.[19] Criminal penalties for doctors who perform abortions, people who "aid and abet" abortion, pregnant people who self-induce abortion, and criminalization stemming from the extension of personhood to fetuses have all been exercised. There have also been new tactics, including threats of criminal prosecution made against anyone who mails mifepristone and misoprostol, the two-drug regime that can produce abortion in the first ten weeks of pregnancy, used in the majority of abortions in the United States. A freedom as presumably sacrosanct as the freedom of movement is threatened by state laws criminalizing travel across state lines to obtain abortion care or abetting such travel.

There have also been headline-grabbing novel legal arguments that signal an increase in confidence on the part of ideologue judges to risk airing outlandish legal theories in public. Among the most remarkable of these was that written by James Ho, Judge for the Court of Appeals for the Fifth Circuit, with jurisdiction over parts of Louisiana and all of Mississippi and Texas. In his concurrence with an opinion that rolled back the Covid-era loosening of restrictions on mifepristone Ho wrote that: "Unborn babies are a source of profound joy for those who view them. Expectant parents eagerly share ultrasound photos with loved ones. Friends and family cheer at the sight of an unborn child. Doctors delight in working with their unborn patients — and experience an aesthetic injury when they are aborted."[20] He takes the language of "aesthetic injury" from a decision regarding the injury done to wildlife lovers when the loosening of hunting restrictions leads to the depletion of the populations of animals they like to see in the wild.[21] This logic, and the mind of the person who dared to proffer it, are easy enough to mock. But to stop at mockery misses the opportunity to articulate the aesthetics, both of exultation and of injury, that attend gestation for those for whom those aesthetics are the most relevant. This essay seeks to offer such an account by detailing the sensory reality of gestation.

Given the effacement of gestators in anti-choice politics, policies, and judicial rulings, it is understandable that pro-choice politics would gather around the fight to attain abortion as a necessary condition of individual autonomy for women. I don't intend to criticize this aspect of legal advocacy around reproductive justice. Rather, I want to affirm that a discussion of gestation is available and necessary beyond the terms set by law. In this frame, the ability to discontinue a pregnancy is the floor not the ceiling of reproductive autonomy. The fantasy of fetal separability which underwrites the progressive juridical tradition concedes the primacy of the right of the state. Our entire gestational politics has circulated around these few weeks when a fetus could theoretically survive outside the uterus. A review of this tradition and an assessment of its contemporary status is a powerful example of the profound disconnect between the concerns of people's everyday lives and the understandings that guide the policies that affect them.

This is largely due to life circumstances and political activities that we have been told constitute feminism. In the United States, the movement for women's rights is narrated as a chronology from the individual right of educated women to attain suffrage to Betty Friedan's monumentalizing of the tragedy of the lonely, dependent housewife whose Seven Sisters women's college degree languished to Helen Gurley Brown's financially independent and freewheeling career girl to the focus on women's leadership culminating in a fixation on putting a woman in the White House as president.

Abortion access has been inserted into this frame. Pregnancy termination is one of the necessary steps to making this other kind of body equipped for participation in the public spheres of economy and electoral politics that have been formed around the social role called man. But, the actual history of reproductive healthcare, the story told in Leslie Reagan's book, has looked a lot more like the vision articulated by Loretta Lynn, the musician and stalwart right-wing Trump supporter, in her song "The Pill" (1975). Drawing on her own experience giving birth to six closely spaced children, Lynn sang "every year that's gone by/ another baby's come" but "feeling good comes easy now since I've got the pill."[22] The speaker is certainly independent from the cycles of unwanted gestation, but not to earn money. On the other side of the pill she's found fun, bodily ease, and pleasure. Crucially, this one tool, hormonal birth control, frees her from the physical containment enacted by a husband who, for years, has gone to the bar "crowing how you and your hens play" while she's been at home "holding a couple in my arms" while "another's on its way."[23] The arrival of a pill to inhibit ovulation significantly reorders the power in her marriage because "this chicken's done tore up her nest and I'm ready to make a deal/ And you can't afford to turn it down/ 'Cause you know I've got the pill."[24] The speaker understands that the possibility of recurrent pregnancy is her husband's trump card in the tactical field that is her marriage. The pill frees her from a circumstance in which every instance of "feeling good" is a monthly game of Russian roulette.[25]

This account is in line with the story that historians of abortion tell. This is a long tradition of handing down knowledge that allows women limited control of their fertility. The availability of abortion and other means to control fertility removes a significant weapon from the arsenal of patriarchy. Sex loses its status as weapon, as a site of control. Control of fertility makes the deal-making attendant on potentially reproductive sex more equal. Rather than the history of injury, feminism could affirm this history of mutual aid with the aim of control of your own life.

This legal and political misapprehension of the nature of pregnancy adheres in more basic units of meaning. The very grammar and semantics of pregnancy on the most granular level work against comprehension of the experience. Grammar software flags the word "gestator" as incorrect. The simple active construction: "I gestated" generated few hits and is so inscrutable to algorithms that Google suggests that I may have been trying to type "ingested" instead. Likewise the sentence "I gestated her" is grammatically incorrect and the software suggests "I gestated *to* her" as an alternative. The same software recognizes "I gestated the baby" as correct, but an internet search for this sentence generates just a few hits in subreddits and in response threads of small Facebook groups, suggesting some extra-grammatical inappropriateness of this usage. I wonder why this grammar — "I gestated" — flags as incorrect. Why do the other constructions read as being so awkward and little-used as to produce the algorithmic suspicion that this is not what I mean?

The answer lies in semantics more than in grammar. What is the meaning of the verb: to gestate? Dictionaries offer two basic meanings, the first transitive (meaning requiring a direct object to receive the action). The transitive definition is "(of a female animal) to have a baby developing inside the body"[26] or another dictionary's variation "to carry in the uterus during pregnancy."[27] The second meaning is intransitive (requiring no direct object). The intransitive meaning is: "(of a child or young animal) to develop inside a mother's body"[28] or a variation "to be in the process of gestation," in other words to be gestated.[29] Gestation, in this sense, is something that happens to one's body. So, it seems that the usage "I gestated her" does not violate the rule of the transitive usage, since "her" is the direct object that a transitive verb requires, as in: I nursed her. I chased her. I soothed her.

So the perceived error must have to do with the understanding of the kind of action that the word "gestate," in its transitive usage, performs. This usage signifies the action of being host to something, here a process. Observe the terms that compose the definition. To "have a baby developing inside the body" does not imply action. The term "to carry" here also means to contain; it means, specifically, "to be pregnant with." This is a usage of "carry" distinct from the most common usage, meaning "to support and move" or the closely related meaning "to transport, conduct, or transmit." So "gestate," in its common usage, means the state of having gestation happen inside you. It does not imply that the person who gestates creates something or performs an action. Gestation is a process you are the site of, not something that you do.

Then, as already noted, in its intransitive sense, gestation is something that happened *to* you, the fetus. To gestate, in this sense, is to be gestated, to be acted upon, just as a cake bakes. But who then acts, when gestation occurs? One is either the site of action or the object of action. It would seem that no one performs the act of gestation. But, in fact, the gestator's body alchemizes the amniotic fluid. It is their uterus that expands.

Their glands secrete the necessary hormones. The food and water they ingest sustain the pregnancy. It is their bones that release the calcium to make the stuff of the fetus's body if they don't ingest enough calcium for the fetus's needs. So the question is: if a bodily process is involuntary, if it is something that your body just does, then is it you who is acting? The right to end a pregnancy is, I'm suggesting, tied to the way that action and activity are denied to the gestator on the level of grammar and semantics.

Consider the other intransitive cases of acts of bodily being. First, those of which the subject is the actor: "I am growing." Second, those in which the action is performed within the body of the subject but by another entity: "The tumor grew in my lung." Consider the transitive examples: "I digest my dinner." This isn't a grammatical quibble nor is it a question of recognition for a glorious achievement. Rather, it's a demand to change language to reflect what happens between conception and birth.

I gestated a baby. I gestated her. To have or to carry are different from to do or to make. Also, the embryo and fetus act on the gestator, consuming nutrients, producing and circulating hormones that change the gestator's body. Therefore, in the long run, my children also made me on a chemical level; their activities remade the chemistry and physiology of my body. The grammar and semantics of gestation make doubly unthinkable its essential quality: one of change and a form of action that obliterates the distinction between actor and acted on, between subject and object. Verbs and nouns must be shifted to correctly represent an active process of production that gradually becomes ever more mutual. There is no single actor but rather a dual action. It is an involuntary process that gradually produces a placenta that emits hormones, filters waste, and transfers water, nutrients, and antibodies to a fetal entity that the gestator has also produced. The fetus's body emits hormones that support its own viability. To honor the reality of this system that the gestator's body initiates and supports is to think the fetus as a fetus rather than as a fiction, a projection of political desires. To honor this process is, simply but crucially, to recognize the difference between a fetus and a baby.

On billboards across the United States, the right misrepresents the electrical activity of cardiac cells in a days-old embryo as constituting a beating heart. This and related false claims attribute human characteristics to an embryo, serving the political project of convincing people to regard a clump of cells as equivalent to a human being. These claims certainly redefine what it is to be a person and must be contested on those grounds. They also, however, erase the intricate majesty of the fetus. The electrical impulses are a spontaneous activity of the cardiac cells or cardiomyocytes, that begin to pulse in an irregular way before "[developing] into a coordinated, peristaltic-like motion of the heart tube" that gradually becomes capable of circulating fluid to the developing fetus.[30] This fluid is supplied by a gestator whose hormones have stimulated their body to increase their volume of plasma and red blood cells to meet increased demand. These fetal cardiac cells grow. That growth is not the activity of a human being, of an agent. Rather, it is the expression of a miraculous biological capacity that is both of the body of the gestator and its own order of activity. The interesting and important, yes I say, miraculous element of gestation is this reality: that an organism can produce an entity that it then nurtures as all of the components necessary for the activities of living develop. The embryo that becomes the fetus does not exist without the gestator. Gestation does not exist without the fetus. The miracle of life is obscured by the premature identification of a fetus as a human, a supposed valorization of that entity, and the resulting erasure of the valor of gestation.

This inadequacy of the available terms in which to think about gestation brings to mind the title coinage of Bini Adamczak's essay "On circlusion" published in 2016.[31] In this essay, Adamczak introduces "circlusion" to "denote the antonym of penetration. It refers to the same physical process, but from the opposite perspective. Penetration means pushing something — a shaft or a nipple — into something else — a ring or a tube. Circlusion means pushing something — a ring or a tube — onto something else — a nipple or a shaft. The ring and the tube are rendered active."[32] The introduction of this simple term allows the unraveling of the conceptually intransigent association of penetration with activity and the implied passivity of this thing for which there was not previously a term. The prior namelessness had partitioned bodies into two mutually exclusive kinds: those capable of penetrating and those available to be penetrated. This false understanding has been a substantial part of the denigration that defines feminization. Gestation, like the physical reality made thinkable by the identification of the term "circlusion," is a process of dual action, of necessarily dual action. The gestator and the fetus must both be present for what is happening — gestation — to occur.

This simple statement is disruptive to the politics of fetal personhood but also to a vision of reproductive justice that monumentalizes the independence of women as the horizon of freedom. It is completely understandable that this latter focus has been dominant in the political climate that has developed since *Roe*. The sharpest cruelty of the terms in which gestation and reproductive justice have been described is that it has taken the place of this necessary conversation.

An account of the experience of a gestator separating from a fetus is essential. This structure of relation does not end at birth. The reverberations of that separation in the neonatal, infant, toddler stages and beyond clarify the very terms in which the social world operates. Freud, of course, observed this, but his understanding was partial. How does gestation reorient us to the question of separateness and connection? What politics does this reorientation provoke? When public conversation laser focuses on the question of fetal separateness and the shape of the legitimate rights of the state, such focus precludes discussion of the actual conceptual provocations of the fetus. The nature of fetality is denied investigation.

The fetus is an object defined by transition into another form. The gestator too, has entered into a modified state that renders them materially different than they were before. "The word 'individual,' ... never referred imaginatively to gestators, anyhow," writes Sophie Lewis because gestation is "a co-production, involving less than two but more than one."[33] The gestator and the fetus are, then, a unit in process. This process begins with a unit in which the non-division is a biological and chemical matter: the embryo and fetus in the early stages of development require the body of the gestator to continue to develop. This status grades into a relation of non-division produced by dependency. The fetus at later stages of development still depends on the gestator even as its own biological development has progressed. At no point is it descriptive or ennobling to consider the fetus a separate entity whose thriving could be ensured through the proffer of individual rights. They are part of a unit whose reality is given little public attention, never mind practical support. This status doesn't end at birth. It is still the unit of caretaker and neonate whose wellness as a unit ensures the wellness of each.

The years spent caring for infants and young children are marked by an immersive repetition of intimate acts of care. You spend hours every day with your face pressed against your baby's face. You know every fold and feature of their body. You clean these bodies. You tend them. Emotionally too, you study your child endlessly, trying to ascertain what they need to feel both free and secure, emboldened to try new things but uninjured and not devastated by failure. You are stunned by their constant change, which is most pronounced and precipitous throughout the first two years of life but seems unending.

The writing of this essay has been interrupted significantly by the fact that my younger child, my baby, has been in the pediatric intensive care unit and the emergency room several times in the last six weeks because of recurrent bouts of bronchiolitis. During this period, I have learned to evaluate her breathing, watching for her belly's pulsations, retraction around the ribs, flaring of nostrils, all of which are signs that her bronchioles are too congested and inflamed to allow an adequate flow of oxygen with the pull of her diaphragm alone. At these times, her abdominal muscles and the interstitial muscles of her ribs are all engaged to try to pull the required air into her lungs. When she is suffering, she becomes quiet and still. Her eyes become frightened. Her breaths are too shallow, come too often, and with too much effort. After each bout resolves and I go back to my regular daily activities, I have to recalibrate my mind by suppressing the tug toward my state of hypervigilant attention to her body.

Parenting is witnessing the gradual retreat of their body as they become more and more able to care for themselves and more and more aware that their personhood hinges on their ability to perform these acts. The toddler becomes irate at the suggestion that you might help her zip her coat or try to feed her with a spoon or wash her hands. She can do it. The same toddler comes to you every morning with the most acutely expressed need for you. Every day is composed of them playing at separation and attachment and it is your job to accompany them through these cycles.

Any caregiver experiences the repetition of attachment and separation as the stuff of these years. You weep alone when you return to work and leave them in someone else's care. You weep with other parents after dropping them at nursery school. How can it be that they will enter a whole social field without your protection and a daily itinerary not under your curation? In your bereavement there is some confusion about the social form of "the parent." *Who needs whom?*, you chide yourself as you walk away, wiping away your tears. The craning of necks on the part of parents at pick-up indicates the ferocity of the need to visually confirm that your child has survived another day outside your care. The caregiver lives in a constant state of suturing and reopening the wounds of attachment and separation. The conceptualization of a fetus as separate from a gestator is a grotesque libel against this essential dynamic of being one and being two. It is the long-missed opportunity to bring the understanding of this gestational dynamic into public discussion and therefore prevents its entry into social concern and reflection.

The beauty and poignancy of this relation, both attached and separate, is a playing out of the dynamics of fetal development. The minute a person is placed on your chest, what is happening is no longer your story to tell. You are now at the beginning of a lifelong process of having to consider their perspective, their thoughts and feelings. You are now two, but against the logic of first appearances, it is through that process of becoming two that you become inseparable. This is the most profound truth that is screened out by a singular focus on fetal separateness. If you are the one who will care for this person, their momentous need for you creates a measure of intimacy and connection that far exceeds what existed when you were addressing an unknown part of your body.

The only way to support pregnancy is to support the gestator. The only way to care for the baby that will be the result of gestation is for gestators to be in the best position to care for themselves. The undecidability between the self and the other is the lesson of gestation. And the powerful have no interest in caring for that process. The unity of gestator and fetus that sometimes becomes the project of radical inseparability between a child and her caretaker is a process far beyond the poor powers of the legal system to define or describe. They can't help us. They can't contain the mysteries that gestation and care present. They can't comprehend the life of my body, theirs, or yours. All they can do, have done, is put parameters around or destroy outright the voluntarism that makes gestation miraculous and not disastrous. The conversion of gestation into an issue for others to debate has denied us the opportunity to genuinely and freely explore it as an experience.

Conservative political forces have tried to steal gestation from us and have been substantially successful as a public matter. But, in the small miracles of our own gestations, they will never succeed. And what can these small miracles offer beyond personal experience? What political concepts and activities flow from gestation? If we were to allow ourselves, for a moment, to imagine a politics wholly disengaged from the terms set by a cabal of self-interested doctors in the mid-nineteenth century, what might those politics be?

It was Plato's creation, the character Diotima of Mantinea, who said that people have children because "they are all in love with immortality."[34] To view gestation as the intergenerational replication of the same, as the process through which a patrimony of little yous is projected into an infinite future is the inverse of my experience. Rather than celebrating my children as versions of myself, I was destabilized, changed, and remade by my relation with my children. Rather than them being me, I became not myself and this was a very good thing. The inseparability that care produces inducts you into an objective state of not-you that has both its joys and its difficulties.

Becoming not-you is a good introduction to a skill that parenting requires. Rather than the font of all things, you must give all that you can and recognize that you cannot and will not provide them with everything they need. Every parent must welcome the reality that many people will provide to their child throughout life things that they cannot. I recognize, for instance that many people (who are South Asian [*desi*], non-*desi* people of color, Muslims) will provide for my mixed-race *desi* Muslim children in ways that I can't. I must flow with the indeterminacy of what their racial, religious, and cultural lines of alliance and antagonism will be. This will be based on how they look and are looked at. It will also hinge on how they feel and what each of them comes to want from the world.

It is not the child who should be made to fall in line with the you who came before. All the capitalist ethics of inheritance and descent prime us to wholly misunderstand the nature of this relation. Ethics that arise from and are deferential to the true experience of gestation would find social worlds in constant processes of renewal. Obsession with lines of ancestry would be replaced with support for the child's radical singularity and the social worlds to which their singularity contributes and from which it partakes. The fetishization of the past would give way to fidelity to the future as the true method for doing homage to what came before. Fear about the status of kids these days would be replaced with interest in kids these days. All this can originate and flow from the actual reality of gestation, a process that reveals the sociality at the heart of any experience of oneself as an individual.

In the end, gestation is a dawning. There is no threshold, no moment when a fetus becomes a baby. Rather, by minute degrees sentience comes, a little more each moment, each day, each week. This is not a process of a baby arriving. It is a process of a baby differentiating, of one becoming two, by minute degrees. The sensations that mark this transition gradually clarify and differentiate themselves. These sensations are no longer of your body, but of another. The act of imagination becomes a relation. We are left with two people who have been changed.

The process of labor and delivery is the ultimate refutation of the right's presentation of the politics of pregnancy as a question of antagonism between fetus and gestator, as a war waged between individuals with competing rights claims. Birth is your first collaboration with your child. It is the process that marks the definitive end of a period when your care reflects an indistinction between your body and theirs and the beginning of a period in which that distinction is marked by physical distance. You have become two. Now separate, you have become inseparable, bound by dependency and care. If the gestator will be a primary caretaker of this child, birth initiates the parent–child relationship as an elaborate collaboration of years.

We are in an era of renewed state fascism on the policy level and trad wife romanticism on the cultural level that, together, threaten us with the violence of a return to forced gestation and a revalorization of the cultural imperative of the sexual division of domestic labor (the enduring reality of which had at least inspired shame in some quarters for a time). Perhaps in this context, searching for gender freedom beyond the individual may feel too risky. But, I would suggest, a gender politics that valorizes women's independence and thus reinscribes the devaluation of the domestic sphere has not served individual freedom for anyone. Liberals have not been able to articulate a convincing politics of gestation and care. Another articulation is being sought, focusing on the inadequacy of the privatized nuclear family to meet needs and satisfy wants.[35] This politics recognizes that independence and autonomy are collectively produced freedoms, not personal freedoms. Just as gestation teaches that the question of who is one and who is two is not as easy as it may appear.

Two: Is a Cervix Cis?

I cannot understand the function of the
living body
...
except in so far as I am a body
which rises towards the world

— Denise Riley, *Marxism for Infants*

"This letter believes that all bodies are intersexed..."
"A LETTER ABOUT THE NATURE OF THESE
LETTERS"

— Aaron Apps, DEAR HERCULINE

I have no desire to mortify myself.

— Christina Crosby, *A Body, Undone:
Living on After Great Pain*

What happens to the thing that gestates? In the minutes following the birth of my first daughter, our umbilical cord was clamped and I delivered the placenta. With the baby on my chest, skin-to-skin, the obstetrician examined me and told me that the pressure of my baby's head and shoulders had produced a third-degree perineal tear. This kind of tear begins at the posterior of the vagina and proceeds through the perineum into the muscle tissue of the anus. That description might sound serious, but this is not a serious injury. Some degree of vaginal tearing is almost universal and a third-degree tear is common. The lead nurse oversaw the cleaning of my body. Then the doctor returned to stitch up the wound, bringing with her an obstetrics resident. In the hush of the immediate postpartum settling, as my bewildered baby clung to me, I listened as my doctor explained her theory of perineal suture: *start on the vagina side of the tear and stitch toward the anus*. She specified the kind of suture stitch that she favors to achieve the best healing result, modeling the stitch for her resident. He asked questions and was offered the opportunity to practice the suture on my body with my obstetrician's guidance. They passed the suture apparatus between them. "Not like that, more like this," she said to him.

Immediately after birth you are, of course, lying recumbent and so your lines of sight are limited. The room is quiet, composed of the people focused on the new baby (you, your birthing companion, and the nurse assigned to your baby) and everyone else bustling around focused on their own post-delivery jobs (cleaning up, recording your vital signs, chatting). The wet baby is close to your face, so you don't have enough distance to really see her in any complete sense. So, for this immediate stunned period, your primary senses are smell, touch, and hearing.

This sensorial situation extends a quality of labor and delivery that I had not expected. My body became very far from me during those hours, but not in an unpleasant way. My body felt like a bike I was riding or an instrument I was playing. I had something that I needed to do and my physical plant was my tool in this effort. I had to make it perform. The entity making decisions about how to weather the contractions or, eventually, when and how to push seemed distinct from my body.

I experienced this distance in spatial terms. The me that seemed housed in my head, the person making decisions, felt very far from the place where contractions were taking place or the place where the pushing was happening. So, when I thought I felt my daughter crown, I had the immediate impulse to confirm this fact by feeling for her head with my hands. *But*, I thought, *of course, my arms can't reach that far,* which of course they easily could and did. I felt her soft head while her face was still inside my body. Perhaps this disordering of your own bodily scale is the result of the last six weeks of pregnancy in which your belly thoroughly separates the top half of your body from the bottom half. In any case, this alienation of person from bodily form persisted in the immediate postpartum period as I lay in the bed. In this surprising perspectival geography of the birth process and its aftermath, the place where my nose and cheek sensed my baby was another country from the place where these two doctors studied and labored over their suturing.

When the epidural wore off I had my first experience of the particular pain of this kind of tear at what feels like the center of your bodily infrastructure. For the hours following the birth, I was still catheterized. Then following the removal of the catheter, during the first day, a nurse has to help me walk to the bathroom. This is the process regardless of whether you're catheterized during birth. She holds you as you lower yourself onto the toilet, and then stays with you while you pee. The slight contraction of the muscles surrounding the urethra are enough to make the tear hurt badly and the acidic urine stings the wound enough to take your breath away. I used the perineal bottle with a hooked pop-up spout that I'd been advised to purchase, since the one the hospital provides, which has a spout like a dish detergent bottle, doesn't hold enough water and produces a stream that's too strong and imprecise and so both hurts you and doesn't do the job. Every time you need to pee it's an event in the days following vaginal delivery. You learn to time your large doses of over-the-counter painkillers to kick in when you need to go to the bathroom. You learn that the more water you drink, the less concentrated the pee is, and the less it stings, or to use the peri bottle to dilute the urine as you pee.

Your providers warn you about the difficulty of the first bowel movement. Toward the diminution of that pain, the nurses who cycle through shifts include stool softeners with your meds and ask if it has occurred as a part of their regular questioning. It is very painful in the act as the pressure pushes on the sutured wound and also following. It requires painful clean-up since you can only use the peri bottle and then blot, not wipe. If you forget, which muscle memory makes common, and do wipe you immediately understand why it is forbidden. It hurts very badly and can even pull out the stitches.

In my second delivery, my vagina and perineum split open again and along the same line. My obstetrician explained that this is common because the scar tissue is weaker than the unscarred tissue that surround it. "Like a seam," I asked, "it rips along the weakness like a seam?" "Yes," she said, "just like that." But, it's also common, as was the case for me, that the second tear is less severe; I had just a second-degree tear the second time, meaning that it stopped short of the anus. "Because the vagina has already stretched and so had more give?," I asked. "Yes, exactly," she said.

In a normal postpartum course of events, you heal these ragged gashes shockingly quickly. Your body grows itself back together, knitting flesh to flesh cleanly in this area where bacteria is so close to hand, where movement seems so inevitable. This process leaves just a white ghost scar at the center of you in a matter of a few weeks.

In her "critical enmeshment" with the cutting of bodies and their reconstitution, including her own genital surgery, the philosopher Eva Heyward writes:

When I pay my surgeon to cut my penis into a neovagina, I am moving toward myself through myself. As the surgeon

> inserts the scalpel and cuts through the thickness of my tissue, my flesh immediately empurples. For weeks afterward, my groin remains discolored and swollen. ... My cut enacts a regeneration of my bodily boundaries — boundaries redrawn. Through my cut, I brush up against invocations and revelations; my cut is not passive — its very substance (materially and affectively) is generative and plays a significant role in my ongoing materialization. My cut is *of* my body, not the absence of parts of my body. ... my tissues are mutable insofar as they are made of me and propel me to imagine an embodied elsewhere.[1]

Heyward's understanding of remaking a body through choice resonates powerfully with my own experience of aspiring to change my body and achieving that aim. I, too, chose to initiate a process that would change the material of my body. I chose to reorder my tissues and redraw my bodily boundaries. I too needed a doctor to stitch my genitals back together. This process surely inaugurated a new life for me.

The first phase of the recovery process for third-degree perineal tears and vaginoplasty lasts six to eight weeks. In the days following giving birth, I kept a notebook to track all the time-sensitive things that needed to be tracked. In one column, I recorded times and dosages of ibuprofen, acetaminophen, stool softener, and vitamins. I consulted it to find out when I could take more pain meds, waiting for the minute that I could. In another column, I kept track of the timing of the baby's feedings and diapers to ensure that she was adequately fed and hydrated. Reading it now is poignant, bringing back the little hourly victories of endurance and progress that mark recovery. I feel residual relief when I arrive at the point in my list-making at which I started to be able to endure longer stretches between doses of pain pills. I remember vividly forgetting to take more when I was due; how wonderful it was to feel my pain diminishing.

During this time, I learned to use witch hazel-soaked menstrual pads to decrease inflammation and cool the area with the shivery cold and pain-relieving jolt of something that evaporates quickly. You also use ice packs to manage the pain and swelling of your genitals. For me, this phase lasted for about two and a half weeks with the pain lessening a substantial amount after the first week and then a little bit every day that followed. *What is the history of caring for this kind of wound?* I wondered as I learned these rituals in real time. I contemplated the tens of thousands of generations of people bathing their perineal tears in salt water or river water and applying poultices of herbs during these weeks of recovery.

The sutures eventually dissolve in the tear, but in that process, the threads' ends will sometimes stick out and poke at the still-healing wound. It is also, of course, always possible that there is a problem with the stitches, that they have come loose and allowed the wound to reopen beyond its ability to heal. After my second delivery, I had enough acute pain that I suspected one or the other of these problems. Sitting on the toilet, I used a flashlight and a compact mirror to check to see if the stitches had dissolved or if the tear had reopened. I was shocked by what I saw. A suture was, in fact, sticking out of the healing wound and this was the source of the discomfort. This was not the shocking thing. The shocking thing was that, gaping above the puffy red, torn flesh sutured with clear thread that looked like fishing line, my vaginal opening was huge, like a slack mouth. My eyes widened; I gasped and steadied myself by grabbing the side of the sink.

During the three years preceding that moment, I'd undergone two pregnancies. During that period I had twenty OB-GYN visits. I had given birth twice, twenty-two months apart. Previous to that, I'd had dozens of appointments with a fertility doctor that included vaginal exams and medicalized procedures that extracted from (uterine polyp) or put things (embryos) into my body via my vagina. This genital structure had been the focus of a lot of attention, both my attention and the attention of medical providers who then spoke to me about my reproductive structures. And, yet, this part of the body had never been less known to me.

Central to anti-trans culture is the description of genital and chest surgeries as mutilation. The fact is that it's very easy to make frank descriptions of bodily processes sound harsh, scary, and in some essential sense, gratuitous. I chose to submit to a process that would result in the blowing out and stitching back together of my genitals. I was allowed to publicly celebrate the elements of that process that were suited to public attention, namely the babies. For the few months that I was visibly pregnant, I received a lot of attention of various sorts and that was productive of a range of emotions. Every time I left the house with a newborn, I was met with soft celebrations from strangers. Another smaller group of people who I knew better and who had experience with pregnancy asked about the physical components of gestation, labor, and delivery in ways that allowed me to share any details that I wished to share. I was shielded from any impertinent attention to my body. No one felt authorized to discuss my vagina in the way that transphobes regularly describe the bodies of trans people. I both can and cannot imagine what it would be like to have such violations of privacy be authorized in the opinion pages of papers of record and the Twitter accounts of members of Congress. I both understand and will never understand what it is like to be addressed by strangers on the internet who engage in the old misogynist glee of describing women's genitals.

I had always thought that I would have children and had been interested in pregnancy. Because of the material conditions of my life and the economy of the twenty-first century,

I waited until my late thirties to start trying to get pregnant. By this time it became a principal focus of my life. This is an increasingly common reality because of economic factors and expanded insurance coverage for egg freezing, IVF, and other reproductive medicine.

This encounter with my own strange genitals was only the most dramatic instance of a regular feature of my experience over the five years that I was engaged in medicalized conception, pregnancy, labor and delivery, and postpartum processes. Routinely during these years, I was confronted with the sight of my organs and bodily structures on screens. I realized again and again how ideated my body was to me, how little familiarity I had with my organs. Or rather, how little I was obliged to think about my physiological structures. Attention or inattention to the different parts of your body comes in seasons, depending on what the immediate concerns of your life are. Even when I knew the numbers that reflect the operation of this or that organ or structure, I didn't know my body, or think of it, as my shock reflects.

My newly discovered ability to change these structures and their processes was equally impressive. I spent these years shooting hormones deep into my gluteus muscles and shallowly into the fat of my abdomen. I read daily reports on the screen of my phone, quantifying the results of these injections. This parturitional process of being split open and stitched back together was only the culmination of this process of willfully modifying my body that had begun years earlier. These modifications were both hormonal and surgical. These were, objectively, sex modifications.

But, it is not only IVF or pregnancy and birth that includes me in the pantheon of sex change. Everybody modifies their body every day. Many of these modifications are sex modifications. I feel very privileged to have entered adulthood having read Dean Spade's contrast between the realities of trans embodiment and the ideologically laden cis pressures that he encountered when making decisions around that care. I read the text "Dress to kill, fight to win" as a cis queer college student. It would be almost twenty years before I would modify my own body through IVF and pregnancy, but Spade's articulation provided a bottom line that guided my thoughts and behavior in my late teens and twenties. I viewed a capacious commitment to the right to modify your body as an allyship with trans people. Twenty years later, I found new meaning in his words with regard to my own body. I quote at length:

> All of our bodies are modified with regard to gender, whether we seek out surgery or take hormones or not. All of us engage in or have engaged in processes of gender body modification (diets, shaving, exercise regimes, clothing choices, vitamins, birth control. etc) that alter our bodies, just as we've all been subjected to gender related processes that altered our bodies (being fed differently because of our gender, being given or denied proper medical care because of our gender, using dangerous products that are on the market only because of their relationship to gender norms, etc.). The isolating of only some of these processes for critique, while ignoring others, is a classic exercise in domination. ... to put trans people's gender practices under a microscope while maintaining blindness to more familiar and traditional, but no less active and important gender practices of non-trans people, is exactly what the transphobic medical establishment has always done. This is why trans people are required to go through years of bullshit proving and documenting ourselves in order to get gender-related procedures, while non-trans people can alter their gender presentation through normabiding [sic] chest

or genital surgeries and hormones as quickly as they can hand over a credit card.[2]

Pregnancy is part of this more open field for modifications that are interpreted as confirming assigned sex. Modifications are inscrutable if they comport with cis expectations; to wit — gestation. When a person pursues pregnancy, if she is a woman, she is not seen as pursuing gendered body modification. She is, however, pursuing hormonal changes, either via injections or by engaging in activity that stimulates glandular production of hormones. To pursue pregnancy is to hormonally modify one's body.

If she chooses to continue with pregnancy and to give birth vaginally, she is modifying her genitals pretty substantially, as my surprising encounter with my own vagina indicates. This modification, more often than not, requires surgical intervention, stitching, in order to repair the damage wrought by birth. But, even after repair and healing, your genitals are different than they were before.

When someone who is not a woman pursues pregnancy, they are also modifying their bodies. This is seen as remarkable or significant because of the perceived discrepancy between a flat chest, for example, or facial hair and the activity of gestation. A pregnant man seems to be making a remarkable body modification because of a perceived discrepancy between, for instance, his flat chest or facial hair and pregnancy. But, the fact is that all of these characteristics can blend in the same body. Cis women too have various degrees of facial hair and variable sizes and shapes of breasts.

I felt the conceptual loosening of cisness through the process of gestation. What precisely does this feel like? I don't mean that gestation made me feel trans masculine; some people have interpreted my remarks on the subject to mean that I felt some distancing from or diminution of a previously secure sex identity. In fact, as a cis woman, I felt very feminized by gestation. The huge increase in the size of my breasts that occurred starting toward the end of pregnancy, and the daily inflation and deflation that marked every day until I weaned my second baby, made me hyperaware of a part of my body that had occasioned little attention. For example, I hadn't noticed when I developed breasts at age thirteen until I was told that I needed to start wearing a bra when I went to play football with my friends. Even after I was told, the reality of my apparently changed chest wasn't meaningful to me.

This feminization felt something like the opposite of dysphoria, as it is described in the clinical literature and by many people. I don't mean counter-dysphoric; as I said, this reordering of my body was not particularly good or comfortable. Pregnancy didn't produce an alignment between my identity and my body. I didn't find myself experiencing a sense of coming home into a body that had previously felt alien or incomplete. Rather, the process was anti-dysphoric in its non-extremity. It was not a source of distress, but nor was it an experience of jubilation. Or rather, the bodily changes only produced jubilation to the extent that they confirmed the continuance of the pregnancy and were part of my care for my babies. As for the material physical changes — I felt surprised by them. I neither identified with nor revolted against the new configuration of my chest and genitals. The process reinforced an experience of embodiment as an ambivalent agnosticism, a respectful lack of interest in the object that houses me. I think this attitude is very common but undescribed. I noticed my rearranged body and was reinforced in my prior view that it didn't have much to do with me. I could observe my changed sex with an emotionally neutral curiosity. This description might strike the reader as a form of dissociation, I don't know. But, it has been a workable way to live in a world organized by the distinction of assigned sex and a hunger to destroy the feminized.

This description pushes back against the common way in which gender is partitioned in mainstream discussion. We are encouraged to place ourselves on either side of the divide between a normalized majority of people who feel comfortable in their bodies or a tiny trans minority whose particularity is defined by an unbearable discomfort. This specificity and degree of distress is the crucial criterion for accessing transition-related healthcare. Cis people don't need to produce a diagnostic account of their relationship with their body as a prerequisite for attaining sex-changing medical services. The ambivalence that I described as characterizing my attitude toward my body is, in this regard, a privilege. I don't need to have a grand theory of my own body in order to mess around with its functions. I don't need to claim that this theory was present when I was in preschool and will persist until my body becomes dust in order to get my hormone prescription.

Experiences that thrust your body onto the screen of your attention, pregnancy definitely among them, can be deeply personal without being identitarian. The terms we are invited to valorize, for example "comfort in your own body" or "comfort in your own skin" as the bromides go, hinge on the idea that this comfort is produced through identification. In other words, wellness seems to hinge on a self-sameness between your sense of self and your form. But, I propose another good way of dwelling in the body, one in which the objecthood of the body is emphasized rather than denied. It is okay, I propose, to view your body as a thing that you have control over, rather than as an organic source of your selfhood or a riddle that you should solve. Your body can, I suggest, remain a riddle and even one that you are not interested in solving.

Here, in this most saccharinified and little-known experience, where the naturalness of your body is supposedly most forcefully confirmed, I found no such thing. If I felt neither a profound homecoming nor a disidentification, neither gender affirmation nor dysphoria, as it is conventionally defined, what did I feel? I could and did view my own body as a specimen. The strongest quality of the experience was the revelation of the extreme malleability of bodies and the speed with which hormones could produce drastic change. This process began with the IVF treatments. I went through extraordinary measures to modify my body and the way that it operates. This newly revealed truth was the general plasticity of bodies, not a unidirectional or one-time change. My body changed time and time again.

Medicalized conception was just a little something I was doing to my body because I wanted to. I was enabled to do this thing that I wanted to do by the policies of my insurance company, broad social support, and the willingness of medical professionals to help me. With their instruction, I had to tinker with my body to address an incapacity that it had exhibited and that held me back from something that I wanted. My body had disappointed me. I was able to hormonally and surgically modify it so that it satisfied me.

Through the phenomenon of gestation, two new bodies are born, or rather, put into a process of perpetual birth. Neither body remains in a static condition following the monumental transformations of this period. There was another, perhaps seemingly contradictory, implication of my years of medicalized conception, gestation, birth, and postpartum. One that is far less hopeful in its implications. This experience provoked the reinvigoration of a long-standing negative experience of feminization. This is the experience that liberal feminism often refers to as objectification. But here again, the actual experience of gestation clarified this process for me beginning with the very start of IVF treatment. The next section clarifies the dual event: cisness loosened and misogyny reinscribed.

My Years in the Stirrups

The year that I was four, I made the same heinous grimace when anyone tried to take my picture. My family called it *my look*, as in: "Stop doing your look!" or, more recently, "Remember when you ruined every group photo with your look?" In the group shots from that year in the mid-80s my parents, aunts, and grandparents look exasperated and my brothers look sweet and nervous. Recently, when I asked my aunt why she thought I did it, she said that it made sense to her: "I think you started right around the time people started telling you that you were a pretty little girl and that really bugged you." Around the time of that conversation, I told her that my friend Jules was writing a book about the history of trans kids. I asked her whether she thought I had strong ideas about my gender when I was little. "I don't know," she said, "you were always talking to yourself and pretending to be someone else anyway. I think you mostly just wanted people to leave you alone."

I had spent a year looking to the left from a prone position at the inside of my ovaries and uterus, hazily imaged on screens. My gynecologist showed me dye whirling through my fallopian tubes and pointed out a shadow on the ultrasound that was the scar left by the egg that my body had ovulated the month before. This began when my insurance company denied me coverage for IVF treatments. They said that the six months of carefully timed at-home inseminations I'd been conducting with the help of my friend weren't adequate to establish a diagnosis of infertility. So, despite my doctor saying that it was not going to work, I embarked on a year of monthly medicalized intrauterine inseminations to prove I qualified for IVF coverage. This process involved multiple visits to the doctor every month for ultrasounds of my ovaries and uterus, taking pills to encourage the development of multiple egg follicles per cycle, and vial after ruby vial of blood to check that my hormone levels were conducive to achieving pregnancy.

The procedures themselves started with twisting to administer a shot in my own glute to trigger ovulation. "Use a stabbing motion, plunging the whole of the needle into the muscle" the online video guide advised. Then I either called to have the sperm delivered from the bank downtown to the hospital on the Upper East Side, or several times (because of Covid delivery delays), I biked to the bank and then hobbled the thirty-five blocks up First Avenue carrying the CO_2 canister like a milkmaid. Then to the andrology lab on the seventh floor to thaw the sperm and then I carried the thawed vial down to the sixth floor. Then into the stirrups, in goes the speculum to ratchet open my vagina, the nurse practitioner (NP) commenting on whether the look of my cervix indicated imminent ovulation. The NP would draw the purple-dyed sperm into a syringe and insert the catheter, which pinched as it passed my cervix into my uterus; one NP told me to say a prayer at this moment.

There were minor but compounding indignities; an NP repeatedly called me by my partner's name, which was also listed on my chart. Several providers asked if my husband (or once, my hubby) was with me. I spent days in the insurer's automated phone labyrinth. That year required so much time peeing on a stick to check for ovulation or pregnancy, evaluating cervical discharge, and checking my underwear for the early pink bleeding that might indicate success or the later red bleeding that would prove failure.

The relationship between genital structures, reproductive organs, and personal identity has been the focus of a new kind of attention in the past few years. This attention was first occasioned by efforts to use language that does not alienate trans people for concerns attendant to menstruation, pregnancy, and various other medical needs. This effort was then met with a mocking and dismissive response from a small but influential cohort of (mostly) British-based feminists whom critics, myself included, refer to as TERFs (trans exclusionary radical feminists). TERFs rolled their eyes at terms like "people with a cervix" and "people who menstruate," and then made the more cutting claim that this language erases women. This same perspective has resulted in legislative efforts in the UK and the U.S. to eliminate trans healthcare for trans kids and bar trans women from continuing to participate in women's sports. After a year of being obliged to spend so much time thinking about and looking at images of these newly ideologically significant structures and organs, I'm left with the view that bodily experiences create many different kinds of connections that are not ordered by the cis categories that seek to constrain them.

In terms of my body, I felt social feelings, not a welling up of connection to my individual organs and structures, but rather an intensification of melancholy connections with people in my life whose experiences intersected in newly palpable ways with mine. Early in the process I met my friend M at an empty bar in Ridgewood, Queens, on a Sunday afternoon. We got drunk and talked about some problems she was dealing with since having a vaginoplasty the year before. Her fetishizing surgeon (he seemed obsessed with commenting on her attractiveness), had alienated her from her medical care and even from its results. We talked about my frustrations with the medical care I was receiving. We both cried about our vaginas. When I showed up to the IVF how-to class I recognized a transmasculine acquaintance and waved to them across the room. They smiled and we sat next to each other, finding comfort in being together in that straight space. We texted each other a little whenever one of us had news or advice to share. My friend S was my IVF mentor; her first pregnancy revealed she and her husband share a genetic condition and so required her to do genetic screening and IVF. What I felt in my body in this process has been made easier by her help. I sat in the audience while D read a poem that compared the experience of being cat-called in a racist way versus a sexist way, evoking the fine grain of bodily sensation that each experience produces. My butch friend G is the person I was closest to in this process as we talk through logistics and decision-making. With another friend, J, I discussed what she's called "our year in hormones," she taking her estrogen and progesterone for her purposes and I for mine. We compared our experiences of injecting ourselves and the results that these injections produced.

Some of these friends are women, some are not women. Some have the same organs and structures that I have, others do not. Some modify their bodies with the same substances with which I modified my body. We were there together, listening to one another; my body's experience was involved in being able to hear about theirs. My love for these people created a bond that affected how I feel about my body and makes me want to protect theirs. History has created these bonds between and among our bodies and these affinities, for me, are the substance of my sense of sex identity, of what embodiment itself means.

For this reason, my social feelings have been historical too, making me feel kindred not just with the people on the other side of the table, but also on the other side of the page. The experience of that year, both the personal and the collective elements, drew me closer to stories I've read or heard. During my year in the stirrups, I thought a lot about an anonymous person whose story I know from its telling recorded in a nineteenth-century sexological text. This person was very masculine and became so distressed when they became pregnant that they killed themself. In a 1917 issue of the *American Journal of Urology and Sexology*, I read about Loop-the-loop, a New Yorker who was sent by the cops to a doctor for being a fairy in the 1890s.[3] He put her in stirrups and she joyfully told him all about her sex life. She pointed out she had a little vagina, unbothered that he called this structure a rectum, as he used a speculum to ratchet it open for examination. I thought of her when I was being examined in related, but not identical, ways.

In the documentary *Southern Comfort*, I learned about Robert Eads, who died in 1999 of ovarian cancer, which was left untreated because he was, at first, not inclined to seek healthcare in the rural Southern community where he lived, and then, when substantial bleeding forced him to seek care, was repeatedly turned away by OB/GYNs who told him that a trans man's presence in waiting rooms would distress other patients. I felt for his fear, frustration, and rage in the swirl of logistics, blockades, and emotions of my year in the stirrups.[4]

These scraps coalesced into this narrative when, at the height of bad feeling about the relentlessness of the procedures I was needlessly undergoing, I obsessively watched a YouTube video of a seven-year-old Drew Barrymore being interviewed by Johnny Carson after *E.T.* made her a small star. She comes onto the stage and plops herself onto the armchair. From the moment the interview begins, Carson focuses on her physical appearance. After pleasantries she says that something is making it hard for her to talk and pulls a plate out from her mouth and places it on his desk, false front teeth that she says her mom made her wear for interviews and photographs. He asks her if she likes going to the dentist to which she says yes, sort of, explaining her thoughts about the importance of dental hygiene. He first insinuates and then insists she answer whether she likes going to the dentist because she has a crush on him. After forcing her to admit something that had obviously never occurred to her previously, he has her guess the dentist's age as though to underline for the audience that what he's doing is compelling a child to express sexual desire for an adult. Finally, he states his intention to "run off with her" himself. In this interview, each time Carson returns to the only topic he will allow, little Drew's desirability and sexualization, you see her look uncertain, immobilized, uncomfortable, incapable of response. This kid has a lot to say about things in which Carson has no interest. When he asks her about getting the part in *E.T*, she says that when she auditioned, "Steven [Spielberg] was worried that [she] couldn't do awe." "Do you know what awe is?," she asks Carson. He laughs. "It's like this," she gapes her jaw, demonstrating the bodily habit of awe for him in a display of genius. He is unable to respond to this because he can't see this person before him. When he looks at a little girl, all he sees is his own reflection. Childhood is an education in this mediated relation to the most consistently immediate object, your body.

The squirm of that interview calls me into my body in a ghoulish and nauseating way that snakes through that year and all of the bonds it forged and reinforced. For many feminists, including TERFs, the memory of this kind of experience is central to their political understanding. Some then make the leap to suggesting that these experiences adhere solely (and universally) to certain structures — ovaries, uteruses, cervixes. Some view their organs and tissues as some great individual resource in which you can anchor identity. I just don't see it that way and not because I don't notice my body or consider it important, but because, for me, what has counted is the way that my body has related to the different people that I cared for and who have cared for me in that year. Those lines of affiliation and the communal feeling that they produce, run in different ways, organize around different points of contact in our different histories. All include a common relation to the ghoulishness of the Carson interview and nothing is denied the girl in that video by recognizing that the hatred of girls and women on display therein attacks trans girls and women with equal vigor. Nothing is lost by recognizing that misogyny and transphobia are eternally and intrinsically linked, actually consubstantial, forces that punish people for their relation to the feminine. That punishment is activated when you are sexed or sexualized against your will, when having healthcare that focuses on your genitals or have such healthcare withheld. These experiences all relate, in some way, to being the inconvenient person in a family photo. You might be able to access some reprieve by being the right kind of girl or woman, but it's always there, waiting to pin you down anew.

The fierce, determinative bonds stem from a sorority and a siblinghood with those who have been looked at, but not seen. We compare our sensations, pains, embarrassments, losses, desires and understandings. These bonds rescued my time in the stirrups, scrutinizing my organs, listening to my structures described, reading reports quantifying my body's functioning, from the paralysis that feminizing experience can evoke because of this history of having been seen as a certain type of girl and also as a freak. These people who allowed me to see myself in them, who, I think, have given me the gift of seeing themselves in me, have rescued my body from an ideology that fixes me as the mute term in somebody else's self-definition game.

There is no life in this body without these bonds, not for me. It is this orienting understanding of my body that those who seek to make cisness compulsory through anti-trans attacks seek to deny me. Ultimately, years of looking at my organs on screens has rescued them from the mystifying ideology on which misogyny is premised. The cervix is not the threshold to a holy vessel. The hymen is not a mark of morality. These structures are ever-changing biological entities that sometimes function as you wish them to, and sometimes do not. I should know, I've been compelled to study mine quite closely over the last four years.

As I've said, I doggedly pursued and enjoyed both of my pregnancies and births. This does not prevent me, however, from a real identification with people who have been pregnant without wanting to be or who have been denied access to abortion care to end unwanted pregnancies. I can feel very acutely the panic that would stem from this inverted claustrophobia, from being penned in by a process internal to you that would severely affect your life going forward.

Representation is the best that liberal feminism can do to account for why we feel this way, this squirming way, and feel it so enduringly. What politics of the body springs from these refusals? Liberal feminists suggest that it's a mental revision that we require. That we can just change how we feel about things, develop confidence and a better self-image. The emphasis on cultivating self-esteem was crystallized in *Reviving Ophelia*, the 1994 best-selling book of advice for parents with teen daughters, in which the author, a therapist, reports her findings:

> that in spite of the women's movement, which has empowered adult women in some ways, teenage girls today are having a harder time than ever before because of higher levels of violence and sexism. The current crises of adolescence – frequent suicide attempts, dropping out of school and running away from home, teenage pregnancies in unprecedented numbers, and an epidemic of eating disorders – are caused not so much by "dysfunctional families" or incorrect messages from parents as by our media-saturated, lookist, girl-destroying culture.[5]

This account of the conditions of girlhood is strikingly similar to that of contemporary gender critical feminists. They too worry that girls eat too little, self-criticize too much, and self-harm in epidemic numbers. This tendency is cathected to the idea of what they call female sex as an eternal font of suffering. For TERFs, the only way to adequately define and defend against experiences like sexual harassment and rape is to falsely suggest that they arise somehow directly from uteruses and breasts, an understanding that requires refusing the reality of the incidence of harassment and assault of trans women. For them, gestation is a point zero of female embodiment imagined as a set of capacities that sentence women to pain, humiliation, and deprivation.

Objectification doesn't seem to me the right metaphor for describing the way misogyny treats women's bodies. In fact, more objecthood, more objectification is required. That the body is an object is an empirical truth. Viewing your body as an object can be very liberatory, or even connect you to it. This is cutting across a long-held liberal feminist stance against objecthood.

This essay is organized around an account of medicalized conception: the routinized experiences of viewing the unknown territory of my body's interior on screens, extracting blood and injecting hormones for months on end. My aim has been to reflect on the way a year of this hyper-attention to my biological and chemical body oriented me away from a mystified idea of assigned sex. The body does not have to be unchanging to be a foundation of identity. The change can be the point, is the point. Bodies change.

The body doesn't have to be a foundation of identity at all. You can be interested in your body's capacities and limits, its cycles and trajectories without feeling that it holds your truth. You don't need to be disclosive to be free, nor should modesty be imposed from outside the imperative of a person's spirit and inclination. The body can be a font of wisdom or it can just be a thing you're obliged to inhabit or drag around. To be shocked by it can be part of knowing it. To recognize that you don't even really know your own body is, in a sense, to know it. Your body exists in your imagination and you often know less about your own body than those of others, your lovers and your children, for example.

In the four years and two months since I became pregnant with my first child, I have had two menstrual periods. I provoked the first, as I mentioned in the previous essay, by weaning my first baby so that I would ovulate and could pursue my second pregnancy. The second period began last month, as I work toward weaning my second baby. The resumption involves massive changes in the hormonal profile of your body. For me one of the most important signs of change was that my eyes have returned to normal. I no longer have debilitating dry eye. There is also the return of my breasts to roughly their pre-pregnancy size and shape. So, the change is ongoing. The resumption of menstruation is a mark of the end of the postpartum period and for me, now, the end of the process of gestation and its aftermath in general. I'll never do all of this again.

I'm now waiting for my third period in the last four-plus years. A forgotten melancholy has blanketed me. My daily mood fluctuates from an acute emotional dullness to despair. But, strangely this sadness feels instructive, like a time out of the kind of eternal competence and resilience that I feel compelled to project every day and with a new imperative since I've become a parent. In prosaic terms: things affect me more. I'd forgotten this feeling. It's also like a little hormonal window to immediate postpartum, the feeling of being taken up by a chemical low that you can hold at arm's length and understand as chemically produced and yet still feel acutely. It also brings to mind a political feeling, the emotional landscape of sustained political activity, in which the collective authorizes us to feel acutely daily horrors that are usually suppressed. You needn't pretend. Everyone assumes that everyone else holds testimony to these horrors in common with those around them. In this state, ambient sadness can express something large and true.

Marking these hormonal transformations by, for instance, injecting hormones or strategically precipitating the onset of menstruation, teaches you that your desires can determine your biological body in some crucial areas of life. This process led me to appreciate the fact that these bodily capacities, which are often presented as expressions of natural tendencies, can be elected modifications. I looked at this body. There was something I wanted to do with it. There were ways I wished to modify it. I had a lot of support in that effort. Everyone should have the opportunity to do these kinds of bodily projects. Wanting to do them is enough of a reason. Although there were hurdles to my project, these were minimal compared to those often presented to trans people seeking to do something with their hormones or organs. The affirmation of this universal personal freedom is why I have opened myself up to the indignity of having a body in public. I was loath to, believe me.

This essay has, among other things, advocated the disaggregation of all the biological functions and physical structures that essentialists draw together to define the category woman, despite the obvious falseness of that totalizing definition. (Not all women _____.) In that effort it seeks to proclaim something about solidarity. Solidarity is not something given unidirectionally and it is not exchanged. It's a shared recognition that participation in a historical project of freedom is a privilege. This essay is not a case of a cis woman instrumentalizing a valorized and unvalued function of a human body for solidarity with trans women and trans people. This essay is the mark of a freedom that I have been given by a genealogy of trans sociality and bodily practices. If I had not been formed by this communally produced and held knowledge I'm sure that I would have felt trapped by the things that happened to me during this time, both the physical and the social. This history has allowed me to understand my body properly, as a site of choice; this essay is my attempt to reflect and honor that freedom.

Three: The Hydraulics of Provision

today it is all grandiose domestic visions truly

in St Petersburg now Leningrad we have communal kitchens
The cooking is dreadful but we get to meet our friends
— Denise Riley, *Marxism for Infants*

Since November 2020, my body has been a factory. Every month since then, for fifty months at the time of writing, I have either been gestating a baby or nursing one. I have spent nineteen months pregnant and thirty-one months lactating during those four years and two months. These figures may seem formidable on the page, but they represent just two standard single pregnancies and ordinary periods of nursing, so are, in fact, non-extraordinary in both degree and duration.

This essay examines a profound conceptual reordering that occurred during this period, due to these activities. Using the stuff of my body to produce and sustain other bodies shifted my understanding of work — shifted my understanding how? This time made thinkable a labor relation without mediation or, in other words, the dissolving of the labor relation. Life-giving activities were available in themselves, for themselves, rescued from their status as labor. When I performed these activities, more so than anything I've ever done for money or anything I've done to keep a house, I understood why I was doing them. The delicate creatures whose every vital sign I assessed and cataloged were right there showing me the essential nature of providing sustenance.

I call the activity of this period "provision" to particularize it from the broader category of care work. Provision is the work of the variable (but almost always cruelly brief) period before you return to wage work and before your child must go into the care of others. Provision is the interruption of what the poet Anne Boyer calls "ordinary worldliness" and, not so much its demands, but the framing of those demands.[1] Or rather, provision's nature is this interruption and it is too rarely allowed to express that nature.

There are a few defining qualities of this time that bear on its conceptual provocations. First, in the temporary disability of your own postpartum body, the work of provision is, of necessity, directed at the self and the new baby in a parallel fashion. This state of affairs can produce a dissolution between the carer and the cared for. Second, provision interrupts the capitalist ordering of time, transecting the work day, leaking care out of its silos of first morning, late night, and weekend hours that a world organized around work offers us for living. Third and relatedly, provision is interminable, against the clock. This is often presented as one of its most vexing burdens, but what if this dynamiting of the clock is one of provision's richest qualities? In full knowledge of the resistance that this argument will likely produce, I suggest that the frustrated hope of provision indicates a revolutionary horizon. We can find a resource in the melancholy recognition that provision's dissolutions cannot remain. We can use the anguish of recognizing that the work of life will not remain the work of life going forward, to sharpen the demand that yes indeed the activities of life-making should remain uncaptured by work. Our dissatisfaction can have consequence. If we share the hatred that the period of provision inspires in us by revealing the depths of the stupidity of the regular workings of the everyday, if we can communize our lonely rage, what could be accomplished?

Provision is, I offer, a hydraulic social process. By this, I mean that it is a rare activity in which there is an automatic and organic dynamic between demand and supply. It is for this reason that breastfeeding provides provision's metaphor. In breastfeeding demand creates supply. The force of need and want stimulates the production of the substance that satisfies need and want. Breasts calibrate and constantly recalibrate production. The distinction between need and want disintegrates. The recognition of the dignity of want could determine the organization of the structures and processes of what we call society. It is difficult to dare see this reality in a world as it is, in which even the satisfaction of need feels impossible.

A cessation of demand provokes a cessation of supply. The physical mechanism of that production and delivery is a flow that has its own expulsive force. Crucially, breastfeeding is not a symbol, but a representative example of this form of activity. From inside this experience, from a common intimacy with its material life, breastfeeding supplies a critical metaphor. Breastfeeding is the critical metaphor for this form of social activity that arises from need and want, calibrates to the direct satisfaction of need and want, and requires collaboration between those differentially positioned within the system of provision. It requires collaboration and reveals reflection.

Provision is the rare productive activity in which the creation of supply requires care for the producer. Your body simply stops creating if it is not well cared for. In the three days following the birth of my first daughter, as I've described, I became a feral animal with a phantom wound whose exact location I could not find and, therefore, could not tend. I did not eat or sleep and I did not want to eat or sleep. I wanted only to guard my baby, who, sleeping peacefully in the soft safe space of my bed almost all the time, didn't need guarding.

I sniffed the air for threats. I found them everywhere and in no precise place. I was most suspicious of my own inadequacy. Certainly, my hazy instinct told me, if I relinquished my vigilance even for a moment, the baby would be hurt. It would be my weakness that would allow this to happen.

This period was also marked, as I've said, by difficulty with nursing. Gently, my mother explained to me that my instinct to forget myself was causing this problem. My milk wasn't coming in because I wasn't eating and sleeping. The lack of supply meant that the baby was having trouble finding the value in latching. She was becoming frustrated and giving up. The lack of stimulation to my breasts then created further barriers to the development of my supply. My fear that I was dehydrating and starving my baby then further provoked my self-neglect leaving only my dry, ineffective vigilance. I was a system out of balance and so my baby and I were a system out of balance. The atmosphere of poorly understood fear produced this malfunction.

My mother told me I didn't need to be afraid. She told me not to give up. She went out and bought oranges and squeezed a glass of juice by hand for me. She made me a small, unintimidating sandwich and cut it into triangles. She put these things near me where I could smell the freshly squeezed juice and see its pretty color. She told me to shut my eyes and lie down in bed. *You don't have to fall asleep, just shut your eyes.* She said she would hold my baby while I rested. I understood as I never had before that I was her baby and therefore also worthy of care and protection. I drank the juice. I ate the sandwich. I closed my eyes and slept. When I woke up, I went back to trying to nurse my baby. I didn't give up trying. Within twelve hours, the milk came in.

This transmission of provision from my mother to my baby via me is the structure that this essay identifies and seeks to generalize. It is the breaking down of the roles of carer and cared for. This is also a lesson of postpartum. Following vaginal birth, the gestator has a measure of physical vulnerability that mirrors that of the newborn. The same fluid that fills her tiny stomach is weeping out of your vagina. You diaper yourself against this rush of fluid as you diaper the baby. A surprising revelation is that, if your baby has a uterus, sometimes you will find a tiny pin prick of blood in their diaper, the hormones of your body provoking a minuscule shedding of the baby's uterine lining. Also, the blood that you produced pumps through her veins and arteries. You don't need to romanticize this watery state of things; these material facts have their own bodily majesty.

The reordering of time is especially marked in the first months when breastfeeding is required every two hours, but timed from the beginning of each feed so that, in reality, it often occurs every ninety minutes and consumes about twenty to thirty minutes per session. That is, this is true if you are able to be with your baby all day. Your work, then, is never done, but your work is never exactly work at all. Your activity is the objective answer to need or want. Need and want will arise as the result of biological processes and individual drives, unresponsive to (because ignorant of) the needs of any other entity and its supposed logics of efficiency. It is to breastfeeding that I look to understand what is important about this time and activity.

The activities that I call provision allowed me to experience work as the exercise of a capacity, rather than as a process of extraction. I felt relief when I set myself to these truly necessary tasks. It's not that this period of care was easy. It was often difficult. The significant quality is that it was not alienated. This activity allows you to experience the difference between arduousness and alienation. The difference is that there is a point to this activity. Ideally, and for the most part in practice, you want to be doing this labor. And even if you don't, you understand its necessity and meaning.

Provision is a bodily mode of care. The bodily habit of vigilance bends you. Your back strengthens in response to that curve of the spine over a crib. You're formed by the incalculable instances of stooping to pick up, a diaper, a toy, a baby. Over time, you may become lop-sided due to the development of muscles from holding a baby in your non-dominant arm, and after head control is established, on that side's hip, so that you can use your dominant hand and arm to do other things: clean a baby, clean a room. You develop the bodily habit of a particular stillness that sets over you when you pause to listen with the hope that a baby has fallen asleep and will remain so. You're like a deer in the woods who pauses to lift her head in order to perceive the slightest vibration.

These forms of action and cessation of action adjust your body subtly to your new great task. These bodily habits are not symbols, they are working conditions. This is a dialectical investigation. It is a worker's inquiry. But from such inquiries, we can draw concepts that are available as abstractions without losing their essential relation to the reality of the activities from which they are derived. Just as labor, in Marx, is both a real embodied practice and an abstraction that can come back around to meet real labor, if you get my meaning, to clarify the real experience from which its analytic power derives. It is my goal to free such activities from their mystified status as symbols in order that they can be held up to the light and examined from every angle. Rescued from its long history as a symbol, breastfeeding becomes, in this treatment, a practice that produces a concept adequate to abstraction. When the bodily things we discover and describe to one another are viewed with this intention we find in them the stuff of knowing. This is exactly how they strike you as you learn to do them and re-encounter the world from the vantage in which doing them places you.

Ticks, fleas, all manner of scary and skeevy gorgers: metaphors habituate us to understand sucking as a negative process of depletion, a game of winners and losers. Bosses and the politicians who work in their interest are bloodsuckers. Oil rigs suck the life out of the earth and move the viscous liquid along pipelines that then threaten to burst, dispersing the unearthed pollutants into bodies of precious potable water. Vampires are a common metaphor for the bourgeoisie. Marx writes that "Capital is dead labor, that, vampire-like, lives only by sucking living labor, and lives the more, the more labor it sucks." The metaphor extends from the ideation of living versus dead labor to the level of individual bodies. We human proletarians are victim to "the vampire" bourgeois who "will not let go while there remains a single muscle, sinew or drop of blood to be exploited."

And indeed, for those of us who work, these metaphors have explanatory power. Who among us has not felt themself to be a husk, sucked dry by the everyday operations of their workplace? Who among us doesn't see their own spiritual parching mirrored in the eyes of workers in other sectors, in the total disgust of a service worker who has given you the wrong order? But, if Karl Marx had lactated I suggest that a different order of critical metaphor of sucking could have arisen in his political writings. As a person in perpetual pursuit of deep understanding and as a lover of language, I think he would have delighted in the concepts that serious contemplation of the material life of this form of sucking and related experiences would make available to him.

Provision recalibrates you to the nature of sucking and this recalibration brings a set of conceptual and aesthetic realignments. Nursing is the second collaboration with your new baby. Following the first, their rush onto the stage of history, as two bewildered people lying the tiny and unfurling stacked on top of the large and deflating, you are encouraged to bring the baby to your nipple immediately. Both of my babies knew roughly what to do; the sucking reflex is famously, but as with so many famous elements of natal experience still surprisingly, immediate and intense.

Your body first produces colostrum; it may have been leaking out of your breasts for several weeks by the time you give birth. It is thick, bright golden yellow, and full of antibodies and protein. It populates the baby's gut, which had been sterile in utero, with the bacteria necessary to do the work of digestion. Colostrum comes in very small amounts to meet the needs of a baby whose tiny stomach and digestive tract are still full of amniotic fluid. "Don't worry" the wise nurses repeat again and again "her stomach is the size of a marble. It doesn't take much." The newborn sleeps almost all of those first forty hours and the task of getting them to latch and extract a few drops of colostrum is your primary concern. If there is a problem with production or latching, a nurse helps you squeeze colostrum out of your breasts and captures it in a plastic tube, which they then use to feed your baby the quarter teaspoon that you've produced like an orphaned baby animal in a zoo.

The colostrum gradually wanes, thins and lightens as its replaced by a comparatively huge flow of milk, which usually comes in after a few days. This astonishing progression occurs as a result of chemical flows that bridge your body and your baby's. When the baby latches and sucks, your pituitary gland releases prolactin, which stimulates glands in your breasts to produce milk and oxytocin which stimulates the release of milk to the nipple. The physical sensation of sucking also releases oxytocin in the baby's pituitary gland. So it's not only milk that flows and circulates between you, but also hormones and the drunk dum-dum feelings they produce.

The Hydraulics of Provision

It's a hydraulic process operating in the complex hydraulic apparatus of the breast. The smallest units of the apparatus are the alveoli, tiny sacs which, like the pulmonary alveoli, pull material from the bloodstream. The alveoli are the site of the diffusion of fat, sugar, and protein from the blood to produce milk. The clusters of alveoli, arranged like bunches of grapes, compose a lobule and 20–40 lobules compose a lobe, the unit of milk production. In response to oxytocin, muscles around the alveoli contract, pushing milk through a system of ducts into the nipple which is the site of holes through which the milk squirts in every anarchic pattern, like if the holes in a shower head all pointed in different directions.

As a result of this process, your breasts calibrate to the baby's precise need. If you have a hungry baby you make more milk. When your baby experiences a growth spurt, your body responds and supply increases. When, at six months, the baby slowly begins to eat purees on their way to soft and then solid food, your production lessens, adjusting accordingly. Your breasts thus both inflate and drain throughout the day and adjust across the duration of the time that you are breastfeeding. You no longer have a breast size or shape. You might go from a round D cup to a soft B cup and back again throughout the course of a single day. Over the course of the months or years that you're breastfeeding, you lose the thread of what your body is, if you are a small or large-breasted person. If you can't remember how long it's been since you nursed, you feel your breasts for fullness. Different nursing positions stimulate the particular lobes on which that position places the most demand and you go hunting to find the fullness of this or that area of the breast. You feel one and then the other to see which is firm and where. You strategize which nursing position will drain the part of the breast that is full or overfull.

Milk comes in two waves, called let-downs, which ideally both occur every time you nurse. The first let-down produces, as my aunt explained to me, something like skim milk: watery and suited for hydration. The second let-down brings thicker, fattier, more caloric milk. If you don't empty the breast thoroughly, which often involves nursing past a period when the milk stops flowing as you wait for the alveoli to release the second let-down, milk left in the ducts can produce painful blockages. You can trace the tenderness of the breast to the place where you can feel the hard blockage. It can feel like a small marble slipped under your skin or can be deeper in the breast tissue and therefore less discreet and locatable. The build-up of milk behind the blockage often distends the area of the breast where the blockage occurs.

The solution is to begin at the point of blockage and apply pressure pushing toward the nipple along the line of the duct as you nurse or pump. This pressure and motion encourage the milk to break through the blockage. This process hurts, especially if there is a lot of milk built up that can't escape, but the acute pain is relieved instantly when the blockage clears from the duct. Clearing a blocked duct is one of the thousands of tiny profound victories that you experience alone with your body and your baby in the postpartum period. If a clogged duct is left unaddressed, it can become infected, a condition that is called mastitis. The blockage can also occur in the nipple pore producing a visible white dot; this is called a milk bleb. In all cases, both the prevention and the cure are a regularized breastfeeding schedule and taking the time to empty both breasts at every feeding or at least emptying one breast thoroughly and then alternating sides from feed to feed. Avoiding or addressing these impediments to flow takes up a lot of your time and mental space during the months and years of lactation.

It is during these hours devoted to feeding that breastfeeding reveals its next provocation. I have already remarked on the breakdown of the distinction between caretaker and cared for, between want and need that characterize this activity. Here, in the hours, whether you are lactating or using a bottle, the scene of provision pushes the theoretical articulation of separation and attachment that was briefly promised in this book's first essay. The hours spent in constant presence with a neonate, or not merely presence but focus, the vigilance that bleeds into your whole life and sense of self, is a quality that is often presented as a unique species of hardship. You are invited to despair that you lose yourself in this period. But, Sophie Lewis has explained the chemical life of this state of being. You are in a chimeric relation to the child you care for; each of you is chemically producing the other. You are inseparable because together you constitute a system that is necessary for their bare survival. This feedback loop also produces the stuff of the carer's biological body. The relation of this inseparability to the world organized by the demands of capital represents this last lesson of provision.

You are inseparable. Yet, this world as it is, organized around accumulation not need, enthralled by avarice and disparaging of those who do the work of helping things grow, separates you. Friends worried about the indignity of being a cow. But I have enjoyed what is commonly called, and we sardonically called, the breastfeeding journey. The world, however, made it very difficult: 25% of workers who give birth in the United States return to work within two weeks of doing so.[2]

I was three weeks postpartum with my first daughter when I went back to work. My baby and I had just found our way with nursing. I wept in my car as I drove from the space around her tiny body in Queens over the George Washington Bridge to the bewilderment of the Northern New Jersey college campus where I worked. Weeping out the eyes, still weeping amniotic fluid into a pad, I began the high pandemic semester teaching from behind as much of a Covid hazmat suit as I could concoct to protect my baby who was too young to receive the vaccine.

My course load had been increased to four classes a semester by a university president who found in the pandemic an opportunity for slash-and-burn austerity. Those of us who remained took on a fourth class, and our increased labor created the conditions to fire our colleagues. Others generously retired with no fanfare to spare a younger colleague, forgoing any celebration of their decades-long careers. I enforced masking on my students who were miserable as a result. They were often coming from working their shitty jobs where they were also required to mask or caring for elders and kids, driving their often unreliable cars to face faculty who were maxed out and devastated by the explosion of their institution and looming threat of their own unemployment.

I spent the semester running back to my office to set up my electric breast pump every three hours. I spent the semester connecting the tubes to the conical flanges that fit over my breasts and the valves and membranes that produce a simulacrum of a baby's sucking. I wondered if the sound of the pump could be heard in the hallway or in the other offices. I suspected it could. I spent the semester pouring milk from the plastic bottles of the pump into glass jars, worried about bacterial contamination, furtively transporting them through the halls of my department to the shared refrigerator in our faculty kitchen. I sat at my desk calculating the time the milk would be in the cooler if traffic was bad. I spent the semester carrying all of this equipment back and forth to my car at the beginning and end of the day. I spent hours, day and night, worried that I had not sufficiently cleaned the soap residue from all of the crevices of the pump implements and that I would feed my daughter milk tainted by the artificial lemon scent of Joy dish soap.

When the flow was good, I was happy. Several times a week, however, the mechanics of the pump, which are after all different than the mechanics of a baby's mouth, failed to provoke a letdown. This caused despair as my engorged breasts throbbed. Hooked up to this device, I would watch the clock as my class time got closer hoping against hope that I would letdown and have time to fill the container before class. When this didn't happen, I would often experience forcible letdown, the sudden and spontaneous expulsion of milk, soaking two circles through your bra and into your shirt or dress. Forcible letdown would often happen on the drive home from work, when I had interrupted my pumping schedule to be able to feed the baby first thing when I got home.

As soon as I arrived home from teaching, sometimes with a front full of drying milk, I would shower and immediately take my baby to feed her. She had very touchy digestion from her earliest days and so almost every time we nursed after I came home from work, inevitably with breasts on the full side of the spectrum following my commute, she would spit up. Several times a week she would spit up a huge amount of milk in a forcible projectile stream. The first time you see an infant throw up like this, you are shaken and astonished. Ever after, you dread the prospect of it happening again. She would soak herself, soak me, leaving a pool the size of a dinner plate on the floor. Gradually, I learned to go slow and take breaks to aid her digestion, but she was often hungry and insistent. It seemed to me she was also emotionally hungry, affected by this intermittent disappearance of the caregiver who was, at every other time with her.

Even with all of the tactics to aid her digestion, she still often spit up. Then we would end our day in the bath together, washing the milk I'd been producing all day that had spent such a short time in her stomach out of our hair and from behind her ears. I put hot washcloths on the areas of my breasts that were blocked and then tried to nurse through the blockages. The pain of clogged ducts and milk bleps was a large part of the sensorial experience of this period. Then I would put her down to sleep and turn to portioning out milk for my baby's grandmother to feed the baby while I was at work the next day. I would sterilize bottles and pumping equipment and repack them. Then I would finish with a final mopping of the places where her thrown-up milk had dripped into the cracks in the floorboard before collapsing in bed next to her crib.

The economic metaphors are perhaps too obvious. The almost immediate re-entry of my body into wage work was beset with minor but sustained catastrophes. The mark of these catastrophes was first, the mechanization of a process that had previously operated according to a biochemical system of need and its satisfaction. The training of my breasts away from the scene of provision and toward the scene of production led to inevitable malfunctions. These malfunctions, in turn, led to moments of abrupt overproduction that couldn't be readily absorbed. Crises of overproduction led to harm to all involved. The conversion of my body back into a thing that worked on a clock produced blockages in my circuitry of provision.

In these weeks, I transformed from being a factory to also being a worker. The second role was much worse than the first. The hydraulic process of provision was encumbered with blockages, interruptions, and alienations. A body accustomed to operating in response to need and want had been forced to become a body that once again fits life into the margins of work. The body rebelled. My baby's body rebelled. These bodies were suited for life but ill-suited for work. These rebellions, these refusals of the body to operate well under the conditions of forced cessation of provision and resumption of production were the next lesson that breastfeeding taught.

And mine has been, of course, the best-case scenario. At every moment of this indignity, I felt my privilege to be able to engage in this pumping routine. Many people don't have a car that they can rely on to get them to and from work or a work refrigerator to store milk. Most people don't have a private office or permission to sit in it for twenty minutes every three hours working around the web of tubes.

With my second baby, I received a semester of leave from a new job. I pumped very little and nursed on demand. There were none of these malfunctions, but there was isolation and loneliness because there is very little social infrastructure for new parents and new babies.[3] Workplace accommodations for pumping or terms of leave that are inadequate for neonatal care set the limits of our postpartum dreams.

There are certainly worse nightmares. In the first year of my first baby's life there were two substantial crises in the supply chain of infant formula. In February 2022, a Food and Drug Administration (FDA) investigation triggered by both a whistleblower report and consumer complaints found a bacterial contamination in formula produced in the Abbott Nutrition factory in Sturgis, Michigan.[4] The FDA found probable links to four infant illnesses and two deaths, all in the Midwest, stemming from this contamination; seven more deaths were subsequently investigated with no conclusive result. Then, in the following year, an acute formula shortage affected the country. Shelves were empty in most drugstores and grocery stores. A less severe shortage is ongoing at the time of writing, more than three years later.[5]

Again, the cruelty of this convergence of circumstances is perhaps too obvious. The imperative to return to wage work (produced by both cultural and economic pressure) runs into the manifest incompatibility of even those workplaces that allow for breastfeeding with the process of lactation. The impossibility of breastfeeding in most workplaces runs into the unavailability or lethal contamination of formula, the only other substance that babies under six months can safely consume. Another order of wholly unasked questions: what are we supposed to do? Why is it that no one seems to care? How is it that the political and media apparatus produce messages twenty-four hours a day blathering about nonsense when the very ability to sustain the bare life of every single person who is passing into the world is such a minor concern that unless and until you yourself become the caretaker of an infant, you have no impetus to know or care about these matters?

What can we do with this frustration and despair, our loneliness and physical discomfort? What can we learn from noticing all the ways that the world is organized against the work of life? Careful attention to this very work exposes the freedoms of the future. Nestled at the heart of this social occlusion of breastfeeding are its lessons. A whole other world of relations between the entity that produces value and the one that consumes value is possible and indicated. In the preface to this volume, I discussed the early appearance of anti-theft devices on tubs of infant formula. The resistance to a regime of ownership, property protection, and stockholder rights is immanent in this substance. The only use for formula is to nourish children aged zero to one year old. There is no other use for this substance. The intersection of great cost and great need makes the formula so vulnerable to theft, so essentially a stealable substance. Infant formula conceptually devastates exchange. Vulnerability to theft in this world, in this case, is the real metric of the only true form of value.

There is often a precipitous increase in general antagonism between members of a couple following the birth of a second child. The couples therapist that my co-parent and I saw during this period called our experience of this antagonism "textbook." The points of tension are predictable: conflict concerning the apportionment of the constant tasks and care work required to maintain the home and the children is overlaid with too little sleep and too little money. Every person I've known has experienced this heightened tension to some degree.

It's not just the increase (which often feels daunting) of housework and childcare that produces this crisis for the parents. It is also the contrast between the kind, all-consuming and uncomplicated provision, and the housework tasks that are snared in dynamics of gender. Although housework seems to be a pure service provided in the name of love, in reality it operates according to a logic of exchange: its origin is the social incentive for women give men a home; in return men give women mediated access to the necessary wage. More recently, in a social order in which almost all people work for a wage, in exchange for the work of social reproduction, you get to be a woman, a real woman. In other words, you attain a status.

Regardless of the assigned or identified sexes of the people involved, and even regardless of their gendered identities, there is usually a gendered antagonism. A friend put it like this: "if there are two, there is always a dad," by which they meant that there is almost always one who presumes that their needs will continue to come first. There is another who assumes that their needs will not be prioritized.

From the perspective of the gestator, there are additional factors. You are healing. You are physically depleted, literally bled out. The amount of physical involvement with your newborn means that you are also touched out, often making any other form of intimacy unappealing. Gestators often feel themselves to be the object of their partner's anger and frustration. Partners are often angry that the postpartum person, who is of the two often the one more engaged in care work, can't do all the things they used to be able to do. It is much more difficult for one person to provide for two or more young children. The violence of your emotions — the love and the anxiety — makes you mistrust your own anguish and anger in the immediate postpartum period and having experienced the surprising effects of chemicals on feelings you may be permanently suspicious of these extremes. So, you are left alone with this anger.

These thoughts have formed around my iteration of the modes of relation particular to this time. While my iteration is not universal, a profound, disorienting shift is, if not universal, then common to every person I have ever met who's gestated and then cared for a baby. So much of the resentment that descends over caretakers in the years that we have young children is about the fact that we love providing and that love is used against us. Our impulse to provide, to attend to emotional and logistical matters, becomes the presumption that we will care for these areas of life. We are left feeling alone, abandoned in these tasks and the identity that forms around them. This common condition of the early childhood years is often shared among new parents in commiserative talks, but it is not treated as the serious substance of politics or thought.

So, postpartum is a collectively endured particularity. We are giving birth in a society that is sadistically intent on making doing so anathema to social life. Loneliness is a broad social condition; but there is a particular iteration of this condition that severs the individual cultivation of a particular life from life as the tapestry of connection, from life as a social system of collective care of all by all. Our society isolates the new parent and new baby. There is little context and little public space for the hours of just hanging around involved in keeping a newborn alive and well.

For these reasons, I don't say that provision isn't alienating. The clash between the world, your former self, and the demands of this new task is often anguishing. There's a physicality of the anguish. It is not the child or the labor attendant to the child that is the source of anguish. It is not even the partner who so often, as in my case, becomes the emblem of all the ways that you are not considered or cared for.

What is excruciating about postpartum is that it exposes how hostile our society is to necessary work, to life in both its social and biological forms. This is why the birth of a child, and especially the birth of a second child, so often produces a spasm of marital discord. There is no way, it seems, to do battle against an entire social fabric that is meaningfully stacked against you. Rather, you focus on the local instance of that system in the form of your partner.

This problem is not limited to the immediate postpartum period, but can linger and amplify in the years that follow. Both partners are wrung out from work. The work of the home is lonely, alienated, isolated. The fact that we can see clearly how social and economic structures produce these problems doesn't make them any less real and urgent in the moment. Perhaps the disruption of the couple form, the exposure of its limits, its insularity, its boredom is another gift that children can bring.

How can we think through it politically in an effort to end this lonely despair, this alienation at the heart of the matter of the home? What is a materialist politics of provision? Nothing is more widely discussed and less incorporated into the fabric of this country than birth. Nothing illuminates the macabre, obscene deathliness of our social system better than the experience of caring for a newborn. It is gestation's very incompatibility with the world as it is that reveals the indignity of work. It is the failure of our social infrastructure and bureaucracy to foster life that reveals the idiocy of a social order organized around accumulation rather than needs and desires. The material facts of this process could ignite, fortify, or revive solidarities if we could let it. Chief among these is the solidarity of gestation, the process through which care for the self becomes care for another. This is how gestation rescues living from the deathly political forces that claim to speak for life.

What of the networks of knowledge and care that can make gestation and postpartum survivable under dreadful conditions? There is practical purpose in conveying the things that are surprising and important about this process. Because, when it happens to you, you realize that there is no talk about these things. And because afterward you forget. I've tried to gather here the things whispered to a friend over the head of a sleeping baby or sent in a group text while desperately trying to get a newborn to remain awake long enough to nurse.

We can address it by valorizing the social structures of postpartum support, by communizing that process. In the weeks following both of my births, my kids' grandmother, their Nanu, came often to visit. In India, where she was born, and in Pakistan, where she had her first two children, she told me that it is typical for a person to leave her married home and return to her parents' home after giving birth. There, she told me, other people do all the work of care, for the new baby, the postpartum person, and for other children. The postpartum person in recovery has parents, aunts, uncles, cousins, and siblings to take over the work of care. They bring the baby to nurse and when nursing is done, they take the baby away. The family brings food, drink, and company. This period lasts for forty days. This is how a thing is done properly. How I cried after she told me this. She knew what I was feeling. She pitied me for living in a place and time with so little culture of life-making, so little respect for collective sustenance and shared joy. She brought me dal and rice, the only thing I wanted to eat. She cared for my babies and remarked on their beauty and their sweetness. She tried, and succeeded, in bringing to my experience some of that expansive familial tradition.

All parents, but especially solo parents, need communal support. Toni Morrison, who divorced her husband while pregnant with her second child, offers an instructive example of a model that reflects the essentially collective project of keeping children alive and well. In the preface to her 1973 novel *Sula* she writes that she:

> was living in Queens while I wrote *Sula*, commuting to Manhattan to an office job, leaving my children to childminders and the public school in the fall and winter, to my parents in the summer, and was so strapped for money that the condition moved from debilitating stress to hilarity. Every rent payment was an event; every shopping trip a triumph of caution over the reckless purchase of a staple. The best news was that this was the condition of every other single/separated female parent I knew. The things we traded! Time, food, money, clothes, laughter, memory — and daring. Daring especially, because in the late sixties, with so many dead, detained, or silenced, there could be no turning back simply because there was no "back" back there. Cut adrift, so to speak, we found it possible to think up things, try things, explore. Use what was known and tried and investigate what was not. Write a play, form a theater company, design clothes, write fiction unencumbered by other people's expectations. Nobody was minding us, so we minded ourselves.[6]

What would it look like if this skill set of sharing things were developed and chosen, absent the harsh imperatives that produced it and still produce it? How can we cultivate an ethos of hilarity and daring, while also making staples widely available? Perhaps these questions are not useful, naively utopian, too unmoored from the daily realities this world. But, at a truly low point in the history of this world, characterized by the funding of genocide and the closing of libraries, can we try articulating what a good life would be?

The period of provision reoriented me to the political geography of the world. All of a sudden, when my first daughter started to walk, the scrap of wooded glen in the park next to our Queens apartment became a precious resource. We visit the roots. We knock on the trunks and ask the trees if the fairies are home. When the neighborhood hawk alights on a tree you can always tell, because all the neighbors gather in craning groups on the sidewalk. As soon as (almost never now, in our poisoned, warming world) the snow falls, children pour out from every building, running to the neighborhood's only sleddable hill with industrial baking sheets and plastic sleds that the bodegas stock to bring out on these ever rarer occasions. My bedtime stories are about a family of rabbits that live under the park. My toddler loves that scant acre of public land more than any aristocrat ever loved his estate. Our branch of the Queens Public Library with its dirty carpet is a palace beautiful. The plastic play kitchen has a pizza cut in quarters with only three slices remaining, the fourth quarter presumably secreted away in some other toddler's pocket. This plastic toy pizza is a beloved object. What paltry rations we are given, these scraps that remain of something called a public sphere. These are the patches of New York City uncolonized by the imperative for maximum capital extraction. They are shrinking. The space for living is almost nothing at all.

How can we think conceptually about the implications of identifying provision? We cannot rely on orthodox Marxism for the answer. Rather, an adequate theory of provision offers a materialist provincializing of Marxism. For Karl Marx, production is the process wherein labor is added to raw materials and tools to produce surplus value. Social relations of production structure that process, as those between boss and employee or among co-workers. Marx deems the recognition of the true historical character of these relationships as the first necessary revision of understanding required for revolutionary consciousness. Chief among these historically produced relations is the one among workers, both in individual workplaces and across all sectors and borders.

In a brief passage of *Capital*, volume 1, Marx acknowledges the role that domestic labors play in reproducing the worker for work each day and therefore reproducing the working class for its role in production:

> The capital given in return for labour-power is converted into means of subsistence which have to be consumed to reproduce the muscles, nerves, bones, and brains of existing workers, and to bring new workers into existence. Within the limits of what is absolutely necessary, therefore, the individual consumption of the working class is the reconversion of the means of subsistence given by capital in return for labour-power into fresh labour-power which capital is then again able to exploit. It is the production and reproduction of the capitalist's most indispensable means of production: the worker. The individual consumption of the worker, whether it occurs inside or outside the workshop, inside or outside the labour process, remains an aspect of the production and reproduction of capital, just as the cleaning of machinery does, whether it is done during the process, or when intervals in that process permit. The fact that the worker performs acts of individual consumption in his own interest, and not to pleasure the capitalist, is something entirely irrelevant to the matter. The consumption of food by a beast of burden does not become any less a necessary aspect of the production process because the beast enjoys what it eats. The maintenance and reproduction of the working class remains a necessary condition for the reproduction of capital. But the capitalist may safely leave this to the worker's drives for self-preservation and propagation.[7]

The process through which the things workers buy become food and the activities that produce "the necessary [conditions]" for the reproduction of the worker remain unarticulated. This occlusion of cooking, cleaning, and care work gives rise to a tradition of socialist feminist analysis that fills in those blanks bringing domestic work into materialist thought.

By all indications, Karl Marx loved his children and was delighted by them. I'm sure he would have wanted to care for them. If he had participated in the care of children, perhaps the necessity of further theoretical elaboration of the "maintenance and reproduction of the working class" would have been obvious to him. It is such an elaboration that grows from the traditions of care that I'm advocating.

Jenny von Westphalen gave birth to seven children with Karl Marx. An unnamed child died at birth. Jenny Eveline Frances and Henry Edward Guy both died just after their first birthdays. Charles Louis Henry Edgar died at age eight. Her three daughters who survived to adulthood all became notable socialist intellectuals. Jenny Caroline died of bladder cancer aged thirty-eight after herself being pregnant almost every year of her marriage from 1872 until her death in 1883; several of her children also died in the first years of life. At the age of forty-two, Eleanor swallowed cyanide after learning that her longtime partner, to whom she'd remained unmarried out of mutual principle, had secretly married another woman. Laura died in a suicide pact with her husband at sixty-six, fearing old age and debility while experiencing political persecution and the economic precarity born of a life devoted to communism.[8]

To read this series of facts produces in me a similar feeling to reading accounts of children's hair getting caught in industrial looms and being pulled out by the roots. It recalls accounts of black lung slowly suffocating coal miners and limbs lost in slaughterhouse work. The suffering of this one woman, Jenny Marx, through the gestation and loss of so many children was a working condition and it cried out for political analysis and response. Advances in medicine and social welfare measures have lessened the incidence of gestational and early childhood death, although these outcomes remain substantially disparate by race and class. But, this is like the innovation of safer looms, not the production of a collective consciousness that seeks to reorient weavers to one another and to the practice of industrial weaving.

Marx calls the process through which innovations in labor are incorporated into the operation of capital real subsumption. Provision is anti-subsumption; it is a social form of production that effaces the labor form. Its activities distract us from work and provoke us to steal away. Like labor organizing or other forms of proletarian struggle, the period of provision provides a time in which we can develop social relations of resistance. It is a productive paradigm for the end of production. This does not happen organically or inevitably, as proven by the last 500 years of human history, in which gestation and provision have consistently occurred while capitalism has continually expanded its reach. This is an aspirational horizon, a message from a possible future and a paradigm for a means to produce that future. Just as shared consciousness of working conditions is solidarity, is a revolutionary necessity and worthy of valorizing, so the work of provision offers a productive feeling, an inkling and an indication.

It is my heresy to suggest that the non-reciprocal nature of provision is the key to its radical potential. Nothing is exchanged. The skills that provision demands are the skills of life. I think this is some of what Toni Morrison means when she said, during an interview with Bill Moyers in 1990 that:

> There was something so valuable about what happened when one became a mother. For me it was the most liberating thing that ever happened to me. ... Liberating because

the demands that children make are not the demands of a normal "other." The children's demands on me were things that nobody else ever asked me to do. To be a good manager. To have a sense of humor. To deliver something that somebody could use. And they were not interested in all the things that other people were interested in. ... Somehow all of the baggage that I had accumulated as a person about what was valuable just fell away. I could not only be me — whatever that was — but somebody actually needed me to be that. ... If you listen to them, somehow you are able to free yourself from baggage and vanity and all sorts of things, and deliver a better self, one that you like. The person that was in me that I liked best was the one my children seemed to want.[9]

Ever since I found out I was pregnant the first time, I hoped that Morrison's description would prove true for me. Nothing that I've read about children rings truer. The work of childcare requires the development of necessary skills and can free you from "baggage" including, for me, that associated with gender expectations. What, for instance, is the status of writing and other art in relation to the work of provision? Toni Morrison provides the following description of a memorable moment when she was writing *The Bluest Eye*:

I remember this more than I remember the book — while I was writing, and I write with a pencil and legal pads, my son is doing something over here and he spits up some orange juice or something right on my manuscript, and I, being a writer, wrote around it. It was so clear. I can always get rid of a stain, just wipe it up. But that sentence might not come back.[10]

Care and thought, care and other forms of creative activity, are not at odds. It's just that our current mode of social organization puts them at odds. Caring for children compels total surrender to another order of perception, theirs. As Morrison writes, this activity requires a degree of ingenuity that is unprecedented in my experience. It's reputation as boring, repetitive, and frustrating work stems, in my view, from its sequester in the private home. I see the difficult combination of emotional difficulty and physical containment in the harried faces of other parents and in the mirror. The introduction of a shockingly small amount of socialization changes my relation to this work. I can live for a week on an afternoon at the park, caring for the children collectively or a morning doing mutual aid with our neighbors in which everyone ensures that all the kids are safe and cared for.

Provision teaches us connection and cohesion, but it also teaches us separation. Even after we got the hang of it, my first child was indifferent to nursing. From her earliest months, I would nurse by the clock because she often would not exhibit hunger cues. When I abruptly weaned her after her first birthday, she made the transition to drinking cow's milk from a bottle with no indication that she noticed the difference. I weaned her so that I would ovulate, which I had not done during the year that I nursed her; this is a common effect of lactation. The month after I stopped nursing my menstrual cycle restarted and I successfully got pregnant with her little sister.

For a long time, my second baby simply refused to wean. She would turn to me in the night to nurse, and demand to continue well past the point that my breasts were empty because she associates sucking with comfort and the process of falling asleep. When I would break her latch and attempt to get her back to sleep, eyes still closed, lips pursed in a little duck bill, she screamed "mo', mo'" while making the American sign language sign for more, two little hands with fingers gathered together pulsing toward each other frantically. Then, with the force of genuine anguish, she began moving from "mo', mo'" to saying "mine, mine." This child, so mild and joyful in waking life, would attempt to wrestle me back into a breastfeeding position, forcing her hands down the front of my nightgown to grab at my nipples. Finally, resigned and enraged, eyes still shut, she cried into the darkness, simply: "me, me, meeeeeeeee, meeeeeeeeeeee."

Weaning is the last lesson that breastfeeding teaches. It is the momentous unhinging of your body from that of your baby. It is an emblem of taking some of yourself back for yourself, hallelujah, and more's the pity, both. But, as the following essay will examine, the promise of freedom is not only, or even primarily, personal. Weaning is the end of your intimate window on what it feels like when things are produced in response to need and in response to want. As I wean my second baby, I know she doesn't need my breastmilk. She wants it. Nursing provides for her in excess of what is necessary for her to remain alive. In my satisfaction of her want, I'm able to imagine a life, to indeed enable a life, hers, for a short time, in which satisfaction of bare need is not the horizon of daily life. This is a cruel horizon that we've learned to accept. Our lives have shriveled to the meagerness that austerity demands, that austerity proposes as the truly virtuous life. In my mutual practice of provision with my daughters, I'm invited to imagine a social order that satisfies wants. I'm invited to consider that having the things we want — all of the things — is thinkable.

Liberal feminism has invited women to overcome our reduction to biology, to prove that we are more than merely gestators. This politics promises the ability to rise above, to act as individuals, to have our own identities separate from care work. This separation, we are told, will allow us to escape the limitations that history has placed on us as women. But isn't the actual imperative that is privileged and supported to go it alone? What is *more than* this? Nothing. Certainly, there is *other than* this. I do aspire to do things other than care work, and am doing those things and will do those things. (I'm literally doing them right now; this writing is that doing's mark.) But, there is nothing *more than* the work of making each other and there is no *other than* without it first. What if it is this society that is mere and meager in the face of our projects to make each other, including our projects of gestation? Then it is this world that should be changed to suit the needs of the gestator and the caregiver, not the gestator and the caregiver who should be changed to fit the needs of this world. So here I take the risk of talking about these matters, coming close to the matters that have been cloaked in sentimentalism to avoid engaging their legacies of violence, because of what it might offer.

* * *

I'm writing these words while my baby naps and my toddler plays with her baby doll, Rumi Junior. "Mommy, can you swaddle baby RJ? Baby RJ is cold." I pause to swaddle the baby doll. My daughter walks away and lets RJ unspool from the swaddle, crashing onto the ground. She brings her again and again. "Mommy, RJ is hungry. What can she eat? Babies can't eat food. We need to nurse her." Is my daughter trying to tell me that she needs something while she sees me writing these words? Is she working out what it is to provide care versus to need care via her dolly, by placing me in relation to her dolly? She's back. "Can you swaddle her?" I'm writing these words. She asks louder and louder until she's screaming: "CAN. YOU. SWADDLE. RUMI. JUNIOR!?" I pause again to reswaddle my baby's baby doll. Now I come back to the page to record that act.

The toddler's screaming wakes the baby. I nurse her back to sleep. She lies on my chest, and I recline slightly to prevent her from crashing backward and balance my computer on my thighs to write these words: I conceived them. It was difficult and took all my logistical effort and ingenuity. I gestated them. It was active, but largely involuntary, hinging on the chemical and biological alchemy of my glands, organs, and other bodily systems. I'm mothering them. It is a daily series of tiny choices, of millions of voluntary acts. I'm with them and they're with me, producing each other still in this new thing that we're doing together. The holy hush of two people, newly separated and newly inseparable, making mirrored crescents of their bodies every two hours, working together at maintaining life, reflects this relation.

Four: Wars, Wars, Wars; or Swimming in the Waters of the World

Wars, Wars, Wars

This final essay is a recommendation of the exercise that initiated it. In October 2024, I listed the years of my life and plotted the chronology of American bombings, invasions, and military aid to proxy actors that terrorized civilians on that timeline. Then, I roughly coordinated my developmental milestones and memorable childhood experiences with the corresponding moments in war. I tried to learn about the reality of those wars for the people on whose heads the bombs fell and whose homes were invaded on the corresponding day. What were these peers experiencing, for example, at the very moment of my first conscious memory? In that memory, I'm lying on my parents' bed in my childhood home with the windows open in the still-cold early Wisconsin spring gazing at my newborn baby brother in a bright blue onesie, his thumb in his mouth. Then I did the same for the timeline and geography of my mother's life and then that of my maternal grandmother's. This practice of considering my life and lineage in wars revealed two truths: one about particularity and the other about a general condition of life in what poet Ilya Kaminsky calls the "country of money, our great country of money."[1]

This Watery Place

I'll speak to my life's particularity first. Before I understood that I lived in a world, the U.S. waged and funded wars in El Salvador, Nicaragua, Grenada, Angola, and Lebanon. In El Salvador, the United States provided a decade of support to the government of a few oligarchs who had plundered peasant lands and violently suppressed the militant communist organizing that had become general in the country.[2] In Nicaragua, the leftist ousting of a dictator in 1979 prompted the CIA to fund and train the Contras to combat the popularly supported Sandinistas.[3] In Angola, Paul Manafort's lobbying firm assisted the Reagan administration in bolstering the anti-communist UNITA government, prolonging a civil war that resulted in the deaths of hundreds of thousands of Angolans. From 1981 to 1984, American marines patrolled Beirut under the guise of preventing an "Arab war" while Lebanese civilians endured invasions of every kind and the refugee populations in Lebanon suffered most cruelly. In all these cases, the wars were the answer to the question: how do you maintain control of resources in the hands of a privileged few against the will of the many? How do you exclusively serve the interests of those who are absentee, whether they are from that place or know nothing of it, as opposed to the will of those who interact with the land daily, who grew from the air and water of the place? Every action was the real answer to the rhetorical question: *What happens to flesh, bone, and blood when the powerful view every war as a game and every place as a proxy?*

As I learned to hold my head steady, to crawl, to eat solid food, to walk, my age cohort in El Salvador were terrorized by the federal military and police intent on returning control of the country to the hands of those that international capital had ordained. As I was cutting a tooth, using words for the first time, and suffering the sharp pain of toddling falls, my small peers in Nicaragua grew in chaos. In Angola, children were compelled to fight as soldiers in the war that decimated their communities. A month before my second birthday, when I was speaking my first sentences, in Lebanon, in the Sabra and Shatila refugee camp, Lebanese Christian militias, with the support of the Israeli Defense Forces, massacred thousands of Palestinian and Lebanese Shia civilians, mainly children, women, and elders. Victim estimates vary widely because many of the bodies of the dead were bulldozed into mass graves.

Two days after my third birthday, the U.S. invaded the tiny Caribbean nation of Grenada. I learned about this event and its aftermath twenty years later from Audre Lorde's essay "Grenada revisited: An interim report."[4] In it, Lorde describes visiting her mother's natal island eleven months before a bloodless coup that deposed the twenty-nine-year regime of an American-supported leader, Sir Eric Gairy, who had entered politics as a leader of a general strike but, in his years in power, moved to the right; the emblem of his rightward shift was his acceptance of a knighthood from Queen Elizabeth II. Lorde describes the three and a half years during which the People's Revolutionary Government (PRG) led the island to retrain its priorities away from the production of commodities for export and the maintenance of the uncultivated land of absentee landlords, and toward the building of health, educational, and transportation programs for Grenadians. This all ended when divisions within the PRG led to an internal power struggle. The United States pounced on the island's instability to invade, an act which ultimately led to the realignment of Grenadian politics between a right-wing and a center-left party who have overseen the island's shift to an extractive tourist economy.

As I study, I try to tease reality out of these wars and the euphemisms used in so-called foreign policy and economic development. I try to piece together what happened. Time and again, sources mention that America's enemies were trying to nationalize industries that had been held in the hands of the very few. Time and again, sources mention that America's foes had massive successes in teaching people to read. I encounter the building of roads and funding of public transport that meets the needs of the people. Building hospitals and medical clinics, dental clinics where there had never been such before, schools: these are intolerable acts. You will observe that this is no expert's account. I'm a neophyte in learning the material life of American wars despite having funded them since I began paying federal income tax at the age of fourteen. Revealing this ghastly misalignment between what I have known and what my money has done is the point of this exercise.

This practice is a way of answering the essential question: how do you study this history of American war at scale? Because, I am advocating the study of war, learning the particulars, the statistics, and the dates. I advocate learning the names of fascists, oligarchs, revolutionaries curdled into despots, and dictators that the U.S. has supported. I'm advocating learning the exact policies proposed and implemented by individuals and groups who had the support of the people but who, not in spite of but because of that support, American foreign policy has deposed or assassinated.

But this is the tip of the iceberg of American history. When you set out to learn the history of American empire, the ongoing history, it's impossible to hold it as an object of thought. This history is so massive and so various. You start trying to learn one aspect of this history and your mind is distracted by other examples. It becomes a question of *what about this, what about that?* Any comprehensive account must begin with the native Caribbean islanders who Columbus maimed and enslaved. But, if you begin there, how can you possibly comprehend the scale of indigenous enslavement and mass murder that occurred in the following years, decades, and centuries on every acre of land from the Caribbean down to the tip of Cape Horn up to the Diomede Islands that stretch across the Bering Strait and from the westernmost point at Cape Alava, Washington, to the easternmost point of Labrador? Then of course, it is not just the people who were killed and the communities that were eliminated from any tangible historical record; it is also the people who never came into being, who were never gestated or born. It is also the communities who were marched at gunpoint and interned on reservations that then became the sites of the most brutal management of the enforced stripping of indigenous lifeways.

If you try to train your mind on the geography of the Americas you commit the obscene omission of the social landscapes of West Africa that were remade by the kidnapping and torture of millions of people whose entire universe of reference (familial, linguistic, cultural) were torn from them in order that they be placed on a far-flung landscape in an incommunicable language to create a lineage population that was instantiated in law and custom as ontologically bound to labor for free. Or the murderous pogroms that have maintained the distinction between legitimate person and immigrant from the first incorporation of these lands into a country to the present day. At every step of these processes, people gestated and labored, and babies took first steps and last breaths.

In this sense, it is impossible to study American war at scale. You could strive to know every statistic, year, date, and famous name without knowing anything about the long history of continual war that the powerful have waged. I studied American war for a time, timing my study around meals so that I wouldn't be too world-sick to eat. And what I learned was that the magnitude of violence disorders scale. If knowing the breadth is impossible, then understanding is served through thorough examination of the individual events. The practice of learning as much as you can about the lives affected, impaired, devastated, or ended by this history is a way of knowing. The fine textures and minor moments of small history are the antidote to the falsity of history as a question of authorities and battles. Recognizing what has not been deemed valuable enough to retain for the historical record is also a way of knowing the truth. When we can't know the fine textures and minor moments, incomplete information, even a simple statement of the number of casualties, still allows us to experience reverence for each life lost if we can imagine each person in the image of those we love.

Audre Lorde describes the United States bombing of a mental hospital as part of its invasion of Grenada. Fifty people were killed in that bombing. Fifty people were killed out of a Grenadian population of 110,000 people. Very little information is available in published sources. I could travel to Grenada to research this event, trace back the history of the institution, discover the people who were killed there to the extent possible, and learn about survivors, if any. That would be the surest way to learn about the meaning of these murders that Americans paid for. But it is also true that, absent these details, simply to recognize that fifty people were killed for no reason other than the maintenance of the impression that the United States is the center of world power is already to know a lot.

I engaged in this exercise, set out on this project of learning my own submerged relation to American war, in order to provide a psychological framework for an experience of my daily life that began when my younger child was around 140 days old. On October 7, 2023, 766 civilians and 373 members of Israeli security forces were killed in the Gaza strip; 251 civilians were abducted. The killings were largely carried out by the Palestinian militant group Hamas with a disputed number of instances of the Israeli military killing civilians and colleagues as they began a military campaign in response. Hamas's enactment of Israel's 9/11, the term Israeli officials and then American media used to describe the day's events, was met with extreme condemnation from across the spectrum of American elected officials and public figures.[5] Weeks of elegiac coverage dominated newspapers and twenty-four-hour cable news programs. The photographs and life stories of the murdered Israeli civilians and those taken hostage were prominently displayed in the media. In many places, including New York City, photos of the victims, captioned with names and ages, were printed and posted on the walls of buildings and the posts of street lights. An atmosphere of public mourning for those killed, with explicit or implicit expressions of support for whatever military response the Netanyahu government announced, was the dominant tone of public response.

This enforcement of selective mourning was predicated on the enforced forgetting of the quotidian nature of murders, disappearances, and internment without judicial process which is the daily reality of life for Palestinians in the occupied territories of Gaza and the West Bank. The shock that the mainstream American public sphere expected to elicit and did elicit from the majority of its population is predicated on viewing civilian death and abduction as exceptional rather than, as they are for Palestinians, routine occurrences.

In the weeks following these murders and abductions, the false claim that Hamas beheaded forty babies during the attacks was highlighted ad nauseum on American media. In public remarks, President Joe Biden went so far as to falsely claim to have personally seen photographs of these beheaded babies. I did not believe this claim when it was first circulated, and yet, it worked on me in some way. It introduced some doubt into my thinking that I didn't articulate and wouldn't have been able to articulate, a doubt that surged when I ran my hands over the head of my baby, when I brushed my toddler's curls. My disgust upon the revelation that it was fabricated whole cloth was intensified by the fact that this lie had snaked its way into my understanding of my children's heads. Who fabricated such abominations? This obvious question was not asked in the media that had been responsible for the circulation of this tremendously consequential lie. Joe Biden was not made to account for his commitment to repeating this fantasy of brutality.

Then in the following weeks and months, the Israeli government began to enact a military campaign to fulfill their widely articulated intention to destroy Gaza and its inhabitants. For many people around the world, myself included, this initiated a daily practice of viewing a genocide unfolding in real time on social media. Every single day for weeks, then months, and then years we saw photographs of the maimed bodies of dead babies and children. We saw videos of children who twitch and cower at the sounds of bombs exploding in the background or from the trauma of living with those sounds and worse every day. We saw photographs of women cradling the dead bodies of their babies, rocking in pain. We learned some of the names of these children and women. We learned the names of the old. We learned the names of men. We learned the names of poets, professors, and doctors. We learned the names of people whose professions did not qualify as worth reporting. We learned nothing of the substance of lives that don't find expression in recognized kin categories or assigned sex.

We learned that children were suffocating to death under piles of rubble, slowly. We learned that children were dying from respiratory infections that were untreatable due to the Israeli blockade of medical supplies. We heard doctors describe the experience of sitting near a child as they slowly died from sepsis that would have been treatable with antibiotics. We learned that doctors were made to amputate the limbs of children without anesthesia. The daily horrors that Palestinians experienced and the portion of that horror that was beamed across the globe to the United States can be fathomed, it can be engaged, it can be absorbed, and this process of absorption can only change your understanding of reality. Like childbirth and neonatal care, absorbing these stories provokes the reconsideration of the vulnerability of bodies and the conditions that keep them alive.

At the time of writing,[6] 50,810 people have been directly killed by the Israeli army; more than half of those are women, children, and elders. In the West Bank, the Israeli state provided arms to Israeli settlers, deputizing civilians to kill Palestinian civilians.[7] Between January 2023 and February 2024, 224 children were killed in the West Bank by Israeli soldiers or deputized settlers.[8] There was no clean water in Gaza. Food and other humanitarian aid is held at the border due to Israel's blockade.[9] Children are dying of starvation.[10] There is almost no baby formula. Malnutrition stems or ends the flow of breast milk for lactating mothers. Mothers feed their infants dates mixed with contaminated water. It's not possible for a baby under six months old to survive without breast milk or formula. Everyone knows this fact, or should. In October 2024, a group of American physicians on the ground in Gaza estimated an indirect death toll of more than 67,413 people due to starvation and lack of access to healthcare for chronic disease as of October 1, 2024.[11]

This wasn't the first time that I came to know about war. Certain stories of certain wars have, of course, been available. How did I come to learn about war? In other words, how did I enter history? What elements became available to me as a child? The year I was in first grade, I had an idea that I thought was brilliant and unprecedented. I assumed no one had ever thought of sneaking out of bed in the middle of the night to watch TV. I used a pair of huge 1970s headphones to prevent waking up my parents. It was thanks to this practice that I sat directly in front of the television, silently and alone, in our dark family room in the middle of the night, watching a holocaust documentary on Wisconsin Public Television. It is difficult to distinguish the images that I remember from that viewing from those that I absorbed subsequently. But my memory, whether actual or amended, is of a face that looks like that of an emaciated corpse, which then blinks. Another memory is of two children, bald and dirty in their striped uniforms, holding hands. I conclusively remember learning that children were killed in the camps. I'm not sure how to analyze the emotional effect of this revelation on me, although many readers of these words probably remember their first exposure to these realities and so can relate. It's a place beyond fear, a dawning of something more saturating and essential about the nature of the world rather than the fate of the self. In the morning, I walked into the kitchen to give my mom a test: "Do grown-ups ever kill kids?"

I didn't tell her why I was asking and I don't remember her response, but it was shortly after this horrifying experience and on the night of my first ever sleepover that I first had a nightmare that would repeat periodically, once a year at first and then once every few years until I was in graduate school. I haven't had the dream in fifteen years. In the dream, Nazi soldiers dressed with recognizable aesthetic profiles (I vividly remember the ridiculous little Hitler mustaches, peaked hats, calf-length boots, and swastika armbands; again, who knows if my brain edited the details in as I grew older) streamed into our split-level house by both the side and front door while I hid behind our cream-colored 1980s couch. They dragged me out by the ankles and handed me a hammer. A Nazi then came in with a baby on his hip and told me I either had to smash the baby's face in with the hammer or they would kill my whole family who always remained off-stage in the dream. That first time I had this dream, at the point of being handed the baby, I realized that I was dreaming and screamed at myself to wake up, which I did, sitting bolt upright in bed. I then walked down the hall of my friend's house and sat on the floor of her parents' bedroom until the light dawned and they woke to find me sitting there. I never remembered how the subsequent dreams ended, but I don't remember ever killing the baby or seeing my family being killed. Until my early thirties, I would wake knowing that I'd had this dream again without the full details being available to me. I was always a child in the dream.

This dream first came to a child who couldn't absorb violence without worrying that she might be forced to perpetrate it. The real nightmare, the recurring nightmare, was about being forced to do harm under threat of your loved ones being harmed. My unconscious had already staged for my young psyche the question that is at the heart of this essay: ought you be more invested in the lives of some people than others by virtue of the fact that you love them? If you answer this question in the affirmative, does that mean you love more fully?

I was living in the Bronx in the childhood home of my best friend the summer after I graduated from college, when I was still having my dream from time to time. I would often sit with her grandfather on the front porch after taking the 5 train home from my temp jobs in Manhattan. Her Ari Zaidy, as she called him and I took to calling him, was a Ukrainian immigrant and the only one of her four grandparents — who all survived Nazi death camps as children, who had survived the health effects of their internment — to become an elder. One day after work, I took my place next to him on the porch as I often did. With no preamble or provocation, he told me his story of the murder of his family members in the camp. He had never discussed the experience with my best friend, his grandchild. Perhaps he was trusting me to tell her. He described watching family members being lined up and shot in front of him. He showed me the number tattooed on his arm. He gestured out at the Bronx cul-de-sac where a combination of his great ingenuity and fortitude, his hard work, and 1970s changes to Soviet emigration and American immigration policies had allowed his family to find refuge. I sat with him. I loved him and I absorbed some measure of the lifelong effects of genocide and war.

My mother was gestated in the aftermath of World War Two, as more and more information about the breadth of Nazi atrocities was made available. She became a young adult in the age of the American war in Vietnam and was among those who opposed that war. My grandmother was born in Eastern Russia in the year of the success of the Revolution. In her history of the period, Wendy Goldman describes the banding together into groups of the millions of orphaned children, the *besprizornye*. They roved through the streets together willing to do anything for a piece of bread, clustering around train stations and restaurants. These multitudes were surely composed of children named Olga, Tatiana, Maria, Anastasia, and Alexei, like the famous children of Czar Nicholas whose murders by the Bolsheviks occupy such a central place in the story of the revolution.

In fourth grade, my entry into the contemporary world came via the opening up of a relationship between my life and the country of Iraq. A kid in my class made a shirt with a puff-paint yellow ribbon on it that read *Peace in the Middle East*. Her much older brother was in the National Guard and was deployed in George H.W. Bush's phase of the forever war. She wore her shirt every week. She wore sunglasses with peace sign lenses. She flashed the peace sign in class. She talked about peace every day. There was a place for that sentiment in 1991 in this mostly white rural American town. There was a venue for a child to wish that a war would end in 1991. There was a place for yellow ribbons around trees and front-porch posts in my community, where many teachers and coaches were also in the National Guard. We were closer to the American war in Vietnam during that year than we are to the wars of the early 2000s as I write these words.

People who are around my age, born in the early 1980s, were all inaugurated into adulthood by the experience of the U.S. wars of aggression in Afghanistan and Iraq. I can date my exact entry into adulthood to the moment that I watched Condoleezza Rice say that, if the country didn't mobilize support for the widely unpopular proposal to invade Iraq, than they were accepting the risk of their own nuclear annihilation. "The smoking gun" in the comically juvenile euphemism for Saddam Hussein's invented nuclear arms "could be a mushroom cloud," she threatened us with.[12] Sitting beside my father as we watched the PBS *NewsHour*, I pictured my mother running through the nuclear wasteland of our town. I pictured my neighbors fleeing like the hysterical children who fled a napalm attack in the famous photograph taken in Trang Bang, Vietnam, in 1972. The children are screaming in terror and pain and they are among American soldiers who don't appear to be engaging with them. It seemed impossible that someone would threaten our mothers and neighbors like this without something to go on. We were also told that this military action would do something for Iraqi women and children, letting Islamophobia fill in the blank regarding what they needed saving from.

But still, I opposed the war. I marched against that war. I took to the streets with hundreds of thousands of people who were then kettled into warrens on the main avenues of major cities. I spent my college weekends on buses traveling to these large marches and handing out flyers in front of the student center. And then, after millions of people had been directly or indirectly killed by soldiers operating according to the command of the political class, we discovered that they had lied to us about the mushroom cloud. The American public absorbed that fact and the people who told that lie continued to enjoy lives of golf and painting self-portraits in oil in the bathtub. We funded the murder of millions of people based on a lie and it simply did not matter. Millions of women and children died of this project to save them. I will never recover from that progression of events. I feel that I can't relate to anyone my age who didn't have some iteration of this experience. We are lied to in order to introduce a measure of doubt into our reflex to oppose war. When the lies are revealed, nothing happens.

Amnesia is structural to American liberalism. When Michelle Obama hugged George W. Bush, she participated in wiping away the millions of civilians his whims killed. The tears of the MSNBC pundits when reporting on the so-called "tender age" shelters of the Trump administration, wiped away the reality of the babies and children likewise interned in the Obama years under Barack Obama's policies. Aggressively white, Anglo commentators on CNN and MSNBC who don't speak Arabic or Farsi or Urdu or Pashto comment on the histories of places that live in these languages in sub-Wikipedia-level terms. They translate the reality of war into well-worn stories that flatter white and Western self-regard. There is the laughable suggestion of Arab jealousy of American freedom. These are stories of mysterious old hatreds based on religions rhetorically demoted to superstitions. These are stories of the baffling choices of the colonized to resist colonization, to risk their children fighting against those who are killing their children en masse. These are stories told in the eternal present of racist stereotypes and there is never anyone present in these reports and interviews with the basic historical knowledge to point this out.

Now, belatedly, what is the general condition that this exercise reveals? Simply that no matter what your particular timeline, to be born in the United States is to be born into a bloodbath, proximate and distant, historical and ongoing. To pay one cent in tax, to have one good time, is to contribute materially to the shedding of blood. Every joyful beer, every baby onesie that you purchase, is a tiny cog in the war machine. My aspiration was simply to learn history as the story of the deprivation and wellness of children and caretakers. And once you start to do so you cannot escape the truth of Walter Benjamin's famous aphorism that "the state of emergency," the opportunity that war offers the powerful to engage in unspeakable acts of violence, is a false pretense.[13] "The tradition of the oppressed" teaches us, writes Benjamin, that the state never relinquishes the powers that it claims are cordoned in an exceptional state. This state of the right to unusual violence is, in fact, usual, general, and total.

The unthinkable act of killing a child is always thought and enacted. The claim that such an act is reasonable and necessary is made regularly by people in positions of great power. These acts are committed in the ongoing wars that are never declared or only obliquely declared but constantly waged. Often these deaths are not a matter of killing but rather of letting die. Here are just two examples from recent history. In June 2024, an eight-year-old child died of heat stroke in a car in an Amazon fulfillment center parking lot in Charlotte, North Carolina; her mother had left her there with the air conditioner running because she had to go to work in the center and the child, it's assumed, turned off the air conditioner and couldn't figure out how to turn it back on. The mother was charged with involuntary manslaughter and child abuse.[14] In February 2025, two children died of carbon monoxide poisoning while sleeping with their siblings and mother in a car parked in a parking garage outside of Detroit.[15] The mother had been calling homelessness services in the city repeatedly, trying to get her children into shelter. There are conflicting media accounts about police and prosecutors' plans in response to these deaths.[16]

This essay is about the moments when the war, the state of war that defines my life, peaked through everyday life. I plotted the timeline of my life in American military aggression from Grenada to Gaza. This is an essential way to express the history of this country. The supposed timelessness of conflicts in Muslim-majority countries is the projection of the interminability of our wars. The pointlessness attributed to those conflicts is a projection of the pointlessness of these wars. The suggestion that conflicts parsed as religious, tribal, and sectarian are somehow less rational than those waged in the national interest provides a way for us not to ask: why? Why have we done this and why do we live so poorly to fund this?

This is the partial story of my life in wars. Each of us has such a timeline. The meaning of these wars is the lives they've ended, the streets, holy places, museums, libraries, and parks that no longer exist. The soil we've poisoned remains, as do the untripped explosives that lie in wait to further perpetuate the cult of death. These wars are a more significant cultural fact than any novel, any song, any film, created in the American twentieth and twenty-first centuries. The women whose lives they've ended, made childless or otherwise made terrible, are a far more important measure of women's freedom in our time than all the progress we are encouraged to celebrate. The destruction wrought by these wars is so total that any beauty wilts when revealed as having been beside this obscenity all along.

I remember the imperative of my parents' generation: bring the war home. The total war is now not only in our home, but in our hands, in our beds, in our few moments on the train. If to become an adult is to come to life and death, to understand the meaning of a bomb falling on the place you live, it would seem the news media is peopled by individuals who are not adults, who speak in ways that clearly express that they cannot imagine a bomb falling and crushing the body of their mother or their child. Social media, in contrast, is full of videos created on tiny screens documenting the words of ten-, eleven-, and twelve-year-olds who rage against the destruction of their homes, families, neighborhoods, and schools. These children have been compelled to learn the history of violent displacement and death. There will never be a before to their knowing that adults kill children.

My toddler and I attend a demonstration to place doves with the names of dead children on the door of the offices of a Brooklyn congressperson who supports the war. I select a dove with the name of a baby who has the same name as her little sister, N——, on it. Later that day J—— says to me: "My body is brown. N——'s body is brown. Ammi's body is brown. Your body is not brown," as she sits on the bed after her bath, looking at her legs. "That's right," I say, "you guys are brown and I'm not." She is coming to understand the meaning of this distinction to the way the world distributes bodily violence. She will likely come to understand at some point that, in the broad arc of the last centuries, people like me kill people like her. We will have to look at each other across the chasm that history has created and reproduced in our very bodies. As a mixed-race person and as an American citizen, she will also have to come to her own understanding of what constitutes and defines people like her, in relation to the people in her life who are likewise called to this process, including her little sister.

As I mentioned in the first essay, the baby has been sick often in her second year of life with recurrent bouts of bronchiolitis. This is the constriction of the smallest branches of the lungs' forks, produced by routine viral infection. It is a common experience for babies under two years of age. But, it occasioned six emergency room visits and a four-day stay in the pediatric intensive care unit (PICU) while she got supplemental oxygen. Nurses sprayed saline into her nostrils and then used a machine to aspirate the diluted mucus out of her tiny sinuses every three hours. In this most serious instance, while I was trying to decide whether to take her to the emergency room, her breathing got scarily rapid and shallow. Her eyes were huge with fear. She closed her eyes against the overstimulation of the ambulance and breathed in the oxygen through the mask that I held over her tiny face.

She hated the IV. She hated the nasal prongs. She hated the thick tape that held the nasal prongs to her beautiful cheeks, abrasing them until they bled and leaving scabs for weeks after. She hated being away from her sister and would call her name in between labored breaths of oxygenated air. She would cry with exhaustion, only able to sleep when she'd arrived at the point of true delirium. She did not want to sleep in the hospital crib but rather to lie on my chest a prospect complicated by the always entangled web of tubes delivering oxygen and recording vital signs. She was not allowed to eat solid food during those days in the PICU because of the risk of aspiration and choking, so even though she was fifteen months old, we went back to exclusive breastfeeding. My body had to quickly readjust to the increased demand and I was worried that it wasn't doing so quickly enough. She would often nurse to sleep and then I would slip her off my breast and readjust for a long wakeful night of vigilance. I remained awake for 72 hours. I needed to stay alert to reinsert her nasal prongs into her chapped nostrils and adjust her body for the nurse to offer irrigation and suction with the least disturbance to her sleep possible. I needed to stay alert to watch the number of her pulse oximeter go up and down. I needed to stay alert to panic when its reading dipped below 93% saturation. I needed to stay alert to consult with the ER doctors and nurses who cycled through our room. Then, with my suffering and yet supremely cared for baby fitfully asleep on my chest, my lips to her temple, my phone held over her head, I would scroll through the photographs of other mothers and other babies far away who were dying of lesser malfunctions of the human body than the one that my baby would survive.

For months, when I dreamt, I dreamt of children in pain, scared children, thirsty children. I dreamt of children whose limbs have been crushed by bombs and who lay, made motherless, made only children, made kinless, themselves dying of sepsis. I dreamt of my own children unable to find me. The particular horrors of the war in Gaza bleed into my general fears about losing them. I dreamt of myself without them, of the living death beyond death. Even when recognizing the constitutive relation between them and me that we call *being their mother*, I realize that there is, perhaps, no more deathly figure than the pair composed of mother and child. This is true whether they are positioned as the native goods to be protected or the foreign pair to be saved by bombs dropped on their heads. These are the stakes of rescuing our bodies and theirs from metaphor.

There were two infants murdered on October 7th. A woman who was in labor and on her way to the hospital was shot in the abdomen. Doctors delivered the baby, who was dead. I searched press accounts to try to find out if the mother survived; they didn't mention if the woman survived or died. I assume she died. A bullet piercing a uterus is a very significant injury. The other was a nine-month-old baby shot in her father's arms in their home. Her name was Mila Cohen. We call J——, my older daughter, by the nickname Mila.

Hundreds of Palestinian Milas, J ——, and N —— have been killed by the Israeli military over the past two and a half years, a fraction of the 14,000 children with other names. I paid for their murders. We can and must note the vastly disproportionate scale of these acts of violence, the difference between thirty-eight murdered children and 14,000 murdered children. Yes, and nothing is taken away from that truth or from the political desire for a free Palestine, freed of racist apartheid, freed from the murderous policies that slowly and abruptly kill children in the service of maintaining apartheid by mourning Mila Cohen. Her life was no more or less meaningful, her death no more or less tragic than those of Mila Mohammed Rafiq Abu-Ghali (2 years old), Mila Anas Moeen Al-Shandagly (2 years old), Mila Bilal Mohammed Shehad (2 years old), Mila Kamal Ibrahim Shaheen (2 years old), Mila Jaber Nahid Abu-Jiyab (3 years old) or any of their more than 14,000 Palestinian siblings.

The names of children deemed valuable are known. We are made to know them. There is no way to know 14,000 names. And even if we could, even if we spend years studying the scrolls that stretch across entire city blocks, listing these names, encouraging us to mourn to scale, these children are still dead. They will be dead forever. The world will forever bear the unspeakable, unknowable, incalculable wound of their lost thoughts, their lost enthusiasms, and their lost tenderness. To love one is to love them all. To protect one is to protect them all. The smell of my child is the smell of each of these children. The movement of my children's limbs is the movement of their limbs. When I stoop to pick up my baby, I lift these children. It is in this way that the gestational sensorium grants me entry into the totality that is history.

Swimming in the Waters of the World

In May 2021, at the height of the Covid-19 pandemic and entering the third trimester of my first pregnancy, I drove down along the spine of the East Coast from our small apartment in Queens to my grandparents' empty apartment north of Fort Lauderdale. I would stay for five weeks. Every day

I walked on the beach, swam in the ocean, and researched and composed an essay for a literary studies anthology. After a year of lockdown and a long, cold winter of pregnancy, working mostly from home with virtually no travel outside our neighborhood, the freedom to walk unencumbered by PPE and the panic of accidentally stumbling into a stranger's respiratory droplet zone remade our bodies. This bodily ease became all the more meaningful as I entered the phase of pregnancy when mobility is most important to maintain strength and support a safe and comfortable labor and delivery.

It was during these weeks that I began to detect fetal movement consistently. From the occasional jabs and kick counts described in the first essays, I now felt large smooth movements that would come and go for a large portion of every day and night. The feeling was a vast swirling, the signs of which you could eventually see when I lifted my shirt. The shape of the baby somersaulting under the rippling skin of my abdomen gave some sense of the shape of the baby to come. Looking back now, I consider how mobile she was in utero in those weeks compared with how little she was able to move in the first months after birth. While she was barrel rolling around and around in the watery place of my uterus, she wouldn't roll over on dry land until she was five months old and then only with great effort, without fluidity.

When I swam in the ocean, I felt that the movement of the baby synched with the heave and drop of the ocean itself. The fluid motion that the amnion made available to her body corresponded with the fluid motion that the ocean offered me. Sometimes when the ocean moved my body, her motion would be momentarily lost to me, so closely did it mimic what was happening outside. Then in that static place between the waves, I would again detect its perfect synchronicity. The experience made me weep with trepidatious gratitude for the fact of the pregnancy and for the unknown beauty that it seemed ever more likely with every passing day would arrive safely. This experience of the relation between the inside and the outside of my body attended the recognition of the transitional status of the fetus moving from being a part of me and to being part of the world.

For years, I have taught the classic 1899 feminist novel *The Awakening*. My students always love it. I try to get them to be worked up about Kate Chopin's almost certain Confederate sympathies or to consider the minor characters who are Black women domestic workers and often referred to by the eugenicist terms that indicate their fantasized fraction of "Black blood." But, my students, by and large, can't give up what they feel when Edna Pontelier swims out to sea in the arresting final scene. They relate to her unwillingness to live a life confined and barred from expressing the intensities of her desires. They've often said some variation of: we know that the entire canon of white American literature has been composed against Black people and people of color, but we will take what we want and leave the rest.

I found myself thinking of Edna's death swim when I was swimming out into the Atlantic in May 2021, my almost-baby whirring below me and below the surface of the water, in time with its rhythms. I wasn't feeling suicidal or anything like. Rather, it was the extremity of desire that brought Chopin's heroine to mind. I felt a dawning relentlessness, a refusal of the small, the mean, of all limitations. My previous visit to Florida had been in February 2020 when I met up with my parents. I'd come in part to spend time with my father, who had recently been diagnosed with pulmonary fibrosis, a condition in which the tissue of the lungs gradually hardens, producing more and more labored breathing and less and less oxygen reaching your bloodstream. He would later die of the condition when my first baby, the one swirling underwater, was nine months old. I also came because I had been having so many bureaucratic hurdles to achieving that pregnancy and I needed my mother to comfort me. It was on that little stretch of beach that my mother told me to be patient and train my mind on each daily step. She spoke of my babies as inevitabilities. It would never occur to me that my mother could ever be wrong about such matters, such is my reverence for her maternal competence. So, as soon as she presented them as inevitable, they became inevitable to me also. After that moment, I never truly worried that I wouldn't achieve pregnancy. So, sixteen months later, during my swims, in jubilee on the brink of my long-awaited first birth and in mourning for my father's worsening condition, I gave all my fear and gratitude, all my joy and sadness to the sea.

Death should be like gestation or rather should be its obverse. Death should be a leaving by degrees just as gestation is an arrival by degrees. It should be slow but not interminable. It ought to give the dying and those who surround them a time together, a time of increased intimacy and proximity, of increased involvement in each other's bodies and the small places of daily experience, a return to the amplified material co-production that characterizes your initial gestation. It is a time to study dying together. Death ought to occur at the right moment in the history of your body, at a time at which you might consent to it. It may even be celebratory, but even if not, it is certainly the site of rituals to guide us. The dying person ought to both lead these rituals in the individual instance and follow them in a lineage of the deaths of others that they have participated in previously. Most of all, every living thing has a right to a death that is the site of utmost care. We deserve a last practice that is a collaboration whereby a body is helped to experience its best wellness on each particular day as a person becomes by degrees less and less alive. They are not my stories to tell, but this was the story of my father's death and the father of my children's other parent, which occurred three years earlier.

What would the politics of gestational death be? The reformist answer is simple enough: adequate leave from wage work for care and bereavement. But of course this is not possible in our current economic structure. If a person were to take adequate leave to gestate and care for children and then care for elders through to death, that person would be out of joint with the demands of the workplace. Life — that is to say real life expressed on its actual scale — is too big for work, it's too much. The creation of sectors of low-wage childcare and eldercare workers stabilize this economic reality to everyone's detriment, to everyone's impoverishment and sorrow.

The generalizing of gestational death as a universal right, like most things worth attaining, is a corollary of a revolutionary horizon. We would need to remake social organization at every level to honor that right. Such a goal would also require a reorientation toward debility and capacity. This would mean that learning of a child's disability wouldn't provoke fear of that child's suffering and inability to survive the world, but instead a collective commitment to assessing and meeting that child's specific needs. Illness, the intermittent or permanent debility that all of us experience, could be allowed to interrupt the daily routine until true recovery, true wellness is achieved, or not in the case of chronic illness or permanent disability. Instead, the powerful prioritize punishment. They prioritize the accumulation of wealth for the very few. They prioritize war.

War is a celebration of killing against the possibility of the celebration of death. War is the glee with which many Americans and Israelis took to social media to mock Palestinians by drinking the potable water pouring from the taps of their houses while Gazan children died of thirst. War is the measured tone of American politicians who sanitize and bureaucratize the crushing of children's bodies. War is the site of the enforcement of mass anti-gestational deaths. It is the maintenance of collective terror as the context for the mass of deaths that are likely either too fast or too slow. Genocide is the inverse of gestation. Gestationality is the tense of what could be; it is that which is being made. Genocide is the tense of what could have been, but now will not be, a blank, an erasure that unspools forever.

These days in New York City we encounter people screaming in pain on the streets or in the train most days. People scream from combinations of madness, addiction, deprivation and despair. "What depraved monster could possibly be always happy?," asks Audre Lorde writing from the 1980s, another era of mass despair and deprivation, the forever condition of this place for too many.[17] In the final two months of my second pregnancy, I was persuaded (and was glad to be persuaded) to give up biking to work and took the subway instead, which I'd done very rarely in the three pandemic years previous. Twice during this time, people screamed at me on the train; the first time it lasted for several minutes until I got off the train. The second time it lasted longer and the person followed me into a second subway car. After the doors closed, I sat down and wrapped my arms and torso around my abdomen, positioning my bag as a shield. I considered what part of my body to leave vulnerable to attack. Where am I thickest, I thought? What angle provides the most material for the imagined blade to pierce before reaching my uterus? How can I make you see that, even in my significant fear and even in my primary concern with protecting my body and the part of my body that was pulsing with a necessarily connected but also distinct electrical pulse, my very devotion to that process and to the child who waited at home for the me/ us that was that body, made me care for that person who for some unknowable reason, for some unknowable constellation of circumstances, was menacing me/us?

I wrote this book because I observed that right where I'd been encouraged to imagine the gravest threat to my individual freedom, in my body's unfortunate susceptibility to become pregnant and therefore limit my earning potential, it is just there that I found one of the most crystalline clarifications of collective freedom. My friend Amy said of her baby, R——: "I feel like I've known her since forever and that I will know her forever going forward." I say, "Yes, exactly." It's something on the scale of the eternal that we can access when we contemplate our children. My children's arrival did for me what faith seems to do for many. These arrivals were, in the terms articulated by the Apostle Paul in the Christian New Testament, "the substance of things hoped for, the evidence of things not seen."[18] They orient me to a totality that is both absent and present, ideational and material. Their care is an object of total devotion that enjoins me to certain worthy principles: patience, curiosity, openness, careful observation, self-criticism, and the pursuit of the good.

For me, constitutive of this miracle is that, when I first turned toward my babies, I encountered strangers. The aspiration to know them and provide for them will occupy my attention for the rest of my life. I have not recovered from the shock provoked by this transition from unknown to central, the exposure of the weave in the fabric of familiarity that their arrivals provoked. The wisdom that gestation brought is my inability to ever face another stranger without the memory of this transformation being activated to some degree. The monumental change wrought by the quick reorientation at these two moments of first encounter permeates my understanding of all things. It is my daily practice of engaging the singularity of my children that sustains this impulse to dishonor the category of the stranger.

The fact is that we are not forever. Our bodies, the infrastructure of our sensoria, have emerged in history and will exit history. But our participation in the real movement of history is a kind of forever. We came from something or rather into something that was already happening. We participated and flavored the terms of what will come after. We change and precipitate change in others. History at every level is in process, is gestational.

Another friend, Navyug, texts me: *but can you tell me, what happens when you have a second child? I'm worried. Does the love you feel for your baby fracture? Multiply?* He can't comprehend any increase or division and redistribution of his feeling for his first child as he and his partner Anupreet contemplate a second pregnancy. I tell him there is no addition or subtraction, but a realignment. There is a change; you change, again. You love your second child for being your first child's sibling and vice versa in a way that disrupts the idea of a separation between the two loves. You love the other members of your family for being in relation to each of them. It is not a diminution or an increase. It is a diffusion, like when the sunlight finds a new angle through a prism and sets another part of the room in motion with sparkling color. There is simply another person where there wasn't one before and everything realigns again, now around a dual center.

If the gestational sensorium provokes apparent confusion between self and other, between intimate and stranger, then good. Consider that this is not a confusion, but the revelation of a reality, a beautiful fact of the world. We are of and for each other. We can desire the projection of this fact, revealed in quiet personal moments, in night-time wakings during the months of internal cleaving, in the pre-dawn of postpartum care, onto the level of the social. We can resist resolving the shocking vulnerability of the neonate into a story about our capacity to ensure the safety of *our* children. Care for the most fragile form of life can be a skill that scales up and generalizes to a personal ethos and a collective social principle. Reverence for singularity is simply distinct from the valorization of individualism. To spend days that heap into years devoted to the children you care for is not at odds with your care for all children.

The moments when I first encountered my children are two embers in the hearth of my life. I hope that what I felt when I opened my eyes and turned my head to see my first newborn in her hospital bassinet can guide me forever. This experience is renewed every morning when I encounter them. Their existence is my home fire. Every morning, I hear the light sound of their feet hitting the floor and then the pitter-patter; each has a distinct cadence so I always know which is coming. I whistle so they know where to find me. They stagger into the living room, arms around the neck of a stuffed animal, rubbing their eyes, and run into my arms. One night, I awoke at three am to my toddler sitting alone on the steps of my mother's house mewing like a cat: "I just knew that if I meowed, then you would come and find me," she said.

The era of the phone camera and the online platform as a faux photo album encourages us to try to capture the feeling of these moments. *Look at them!*, our posting practices say ad nauseam to our friends and followers. But babies are blessedly like the moon. Blessedly, the things they manifest in their variously (and anomalously) accented toddler language, their dancing styles that reflect nothing but what the body has to say to music, the fine line between their tenderness and their violence, their essences, in short, are resistant to representation. This is most true of visual representation. The prosaic tiny white circle above the horizon is the analog to even the cutest snapshot of a child. My friend Nada and I never miss the opportunity to send each other the moon. But, the point of our practice is not to show the other what we're seeing.

Rather, the sender counts on the receiver to infuse her reverence for the celestial into what is on the screen, which is always nothing like what the sender sees in real life. This book has been my effort to test the potential of words in this regard and as regards gestation. I have not been so foolish as to think that I could translate my children and their lessons into words. Rather, I have aimed at the more modest goal of evoking your experience with the children in your care. I have hoped to deliver you back to a place that you've been rather than taking you back with me.

I have been split, first into two, then another part of me flaked off, so that now I am three. I decided to have a second baby in large part because I felt that I couldn't sustain the degree of vigilant attention that my first child provoked or more importantly, that this degree of vigilance would be bad for her. I felt I could not endure the force of the singular relation to her. The joke was on me, as my second child has in no way lessened or diffused that force. I'm no less mad with love than I was before. In fact, the moment when one child sees the other in pain or distress and moves toward her sibling to comfort presents a new horizon of unendurable tenderness.

This is a way that people can feel about each other. That is the wonder at the center of this book in the plainest terms. The anguishing conflict between that feeling and the demands of the world is real, but it is not inevitable and it won't be eternal. People made this world and people will make the next. The precise shape that days would take and the way the streets would feel after the reign of the divine right of kings was unimaginable before the guillotines fell. Still, many people did know that something else, something better was possible. How did they know? The people knew because they measured the beauty of the world against the brutality of the powerful. They knew that the sparkle of the empress's crown emeralds was a pathetic simulacrum of the beauty of every green harvest and glades of ferns that spring up where the light dapples through the forest canopy. They knew that the pomp and circumstance was like popular spectacles of torture: both poor derivatives of the people's festivals. They knew their shared stories explained the world, not declarations from on high. They had perhaps felt the care of a friend or the sympathy of a mother. Many knew, in short, what love feels like.

Today, we know the unreality of the noise of the falsely bifurcated political class. We know that their manufactured bickering masks their shared purpose and is a silly distraction from noticing all that we don't have and why, from demanding what we deserve. We know the wealth of this place: the shocking cliffs plunging to the briny Pacific, the natural sulfur hot springs on the Havasupai, the boreal forests growing out of the boundary waters, the living swamps where Maroons liberated each other, and the humic hum of the Everglades. We know that people can squeeze life out of chatting in an exurban all-night donut shop and the small kindness of your kid's teacher noticing something essential about your child. We've seen a librarian stoop down to speak directly to a child and we've gathered with twelve of our neighbors in protest to protect our library from hateful ideologues who want to determine which books we should be allowed to read. All we have are the myriad ways that we help each other when we're all so tired and so sad. We're so angry and so scared. Even now, the watery places are here and we give them to one another.

In New York City, from the heights of Inwood on Manahatta, we see the slow slide of the Muh-he-kun-ne-tuk River and we see the water-formed schist that grants a view of the island's substrata peaking out of the park. We tend the collective memory of kids jumping off this island into the river on a hot August day when we ride the bus to the still-free beaches. We walk the same streets once walked by the girls who were on strike to save each other from misery and death and stumble upon monuments to the city's stops on the underground railroad. We know the glory of the feeling when the song of summer bumps and of being together in the park. That is where we see our neighbors dancing while in the middle of a blanket, at the center of the music and ecstatic partying, attended by everyone's mobile attention, a baby has learned to sleep, cheek to earth, arms gathered beneath her chest, butt in the air. We can convince each other that releasing all these beautiful feelings from their sequester in the few hours we have for each other is not only possible but inevitable. The perpetual pursuit of that release is the only way to keep ourselves and them, in all senses of the word, alive.

Notes

Preface: Us

1. This chapter title is inspired by Sylvia Plath's poem "Daddy," in which the speaker connects her general despair over the despotism of her father and her husband to the fate of "the Polish town/ scraped flat by the roller/ of wars, wars, wars."
2. Sophie Lewis, *Full Surrogacy Now: Feminism Against Family* (London, Verso, 2019), 160.

1 Fetal Separateness

1. United States Supreme Court, *Thomas E. Dobbs, State Health Officer of the Mississippi Department of Health, et al. v. Jackson Women's Health Organization, et al.* (2021), https://www.supremecourt.gov/oral_arguments/argument_transcripts/2021/19-1392_bq7d.pdf, accessed May 8, 2025.
2. Jericka Duncan, Rachel Bailey, Hilary Cook. "Brittany Watts, Ohio women charged with felony after miscarriage at home describes shock of her arrest," *CBS News*, October 21, 2024, https://www.cbsnews.com/news/brittany-watts-the-ohio-woman-charged-with-a-felony-after-a-miscarriage-talks-shock-of-her-arrest/
3. Other priorities of the right reflect aspirations to control fertility before fertilization. These include: contraception denials, forcing doctors to notify parents of minors about contraception prescriptions, and the centrality of reproductive futures to efforts to ban gender affirming.
4. Adrienne Rich, *Of Woman Born: Motherhood as Experience and Institution* (New York, W.W. Norton, 1995), 63.

5. *Roe et al. v. Wade, District Attorney of Dallas County*, 70-18 (1973). Library of Congress, https://tile.loc.gov/storage-services/service/ll/usrep/usrep410/usrep410113/usrep410113.pdf
6. Ibid.
7. Ibid.
8. Ibid.
9. Ibid.
10. Ibid.
11. *Planned Parenthood of Southeastern Pennsylvania v. Casey*, 505 U.S. 833 (1992). Library of Congress, https://www.loc.gov/item/usrep505833/
12. Ibid.
13. *Dobbs v. Jackson Women's Health*, 597 U.S. 215 (2022).
14. Leslie J. Reagan, *When Abortion Was a Crime: Women, Medicine, and Law in the United States, 1867–1973* (Berkeley: University of California Press, 1997).
15. *Dobbs v. Jackson Women's Health*, 597 U.S. 215 (2022).
16. Ibid.
17. Ibid.
18. Ibid.
19. https://www.guttmacher.org/state-policy/explore/state-policies-abortion-bans
20. Susan Rinkunas, "Trump-appointed judge cites wildlife cases as a reason to ban abortion pills," *Jezebel*, April 17, 2023, https://www.jezebel.com/trump-appointed-judge-cites-wildlife-cases-as-a-reason-1850747308
21. Ibid.
22. Loretta Lynn, "The Pill," on *Back to the Country*, MCA Records, 1975.
23. Ibid.
24. Ibid.
25. Ibid.
26. *Cambridge Dictionary*, s.v. gestate (tv), https://dictionary.cambridge.org/us/dictionary/english/gestated, accessed May 9, 2025.

27. *Merriam-Webster*, s.v. gestate (tv), https://www.merriam-webster.com/dictionary/gestate, accessed May 9, 2025.
28. *Cambridge Dictionary*, sv gestate (iv).
29. *Merriam-Webster*, s.v. gestate (iv).
30. Jörg Männer, "When does the human embryonic heart start beating? A review of contemporary and historical sources of knowledge about the onset of blood circulation," *Journal of Cardiovascular Development and Disease*, https://pmc.ncbi.nlm.nih.gov/articles/PMC9225347/, accessed May 9, 2025.
31. Bini Adamczak, "Six years (and counting) of circlusion," trans. Sophie Lewis, *The New Inquiry*, August 22, 2022, https://thenewinquiry.com/six-years-and-counting-of-circlusion/, accessed May 9, 2025.
32. Ibid.
33. Lewis, *Full Surrogacy Now*, p. 160.
34. Plato, "The Symposium," *The Complete Works*, edited by John M. Cooper, trans. Alexander Nehamas and Paul Woodruff (Indianapolis/Cambridge: Hackett Publishing Co., 1997), 491.
35. See M.E. O'Brien, *Family Abolition: Capitalism and the Communizing of Care* (London, Pluto Press, 2023) and Sophie Lewis, *Abolish the Family: A Manifesto for Care and Liberation* (London, Verso, 2022).

2 Is a Cervix Cis?

1. Eva Heyward, "More lessons from a starfish: Prefixial flesh and transpeciated selves," *Women's Studies Quarterly* 36(3/4), Fall–Winter 2008, 64–85.
2. Dean Spade, "Dress to kill, fight to win," *LTTR Journal* #1, September 2002.
3. R.W. Shufeldt, "Biography of a passive pederast," *American Journal of Urology and Sexology* 13, 1917, 451–460.
4. *Southern Comfort*, directed by Kate Davis (HBO Documentary, 2001).

5. Mary Bray Pipher, *Reviving Ophelia: Saving the Selves of Adolescent Girls* (New York, Putnam, 1994).

3 The Hydraulics of Provision

1. Anne Boyer, "At least two types of people," in *Garments Against Women* (Boise, ID, Ahsahta Press, 2015), 23.
2. Kristen Gallant, "The heart-shattering feeling of going back to work after having a baby," *Time*, April 12, 2023, https://time.com/6270034/back-to-work-after-baby-kristin-gallant/, accessed May 10, 2025.
3. This situation will become much worse if we see the continued spread of vaccination resistance. The threat of measles, mumps, rubella, whooping cough, polio and other childhood illnesses that have long been controlled by vaccines would make it dangerous for babies to be in public spaces for the first year of life.
4. Food and Drug Administration Statement, "FDA investigation of Cronobacter infections: Powdered infant formula," February 2022, https://www.fda.gov/food/outbreaks-foodborne-illness/fda-investigation-cronobacter-infections-powdered-infant-formula-february-2022, accessed May 12, 2025.
5. United States Government Accountability Office, "Baby formula's biggest buyer takes a closer look at supplies and shortages," January 15, 2025, https://www.gao.gov/blog/baby-formulas-biggest-buyer-takes-closer-look-supplies-and-shortages, accessed May 12, 2025.
6. Toni Morrison, *Sula* (New York, Knopf Doubleday, 2002), xiv–xv.
7. Karl Marx, *Capital: A Critique of Political Economy*, vol. 1, trans. Ben Fowkes (New York, Penguin, 1992), 717–718.
8. Mary Gabriel, *Love and Capital: Karl and Jenny Marx and the Birth of a Revolution* (New York, Little, Brown, 2011).

9. Bill Moyers, "Toni Morrison on love and writing," March 11, 1990, https://billmoyers.com/content/toni-morrison-part-1/, accessed May 9, 2025.
10. Toni Morrison, "Toni Morrison describes how she began to be a writer," August 14, 2016, https://www.macdowell.org/news/toni-morrison-describes-how-she-began-to-be-a-writer, accessed May 9, 2025.

4 Wars, Wars, Wars; or Swimming in the Waters of the World

1. Ilya Kaminsky, "We lived happily during the war," *Deaf Republic: Poems* (United States: Graywolf Press, 2019), 3.
2. James Dunkerley, "Postscript," in *The Long War: Dictatorship and Revolution in El Salvador* (New York, Verso, 1985), 215–311.
3. Noam Chomsky, *Turning the Tide* (London, Pluto Press, 2015), 117–135.
4. Audre Lorde, "Grenada revisited: An interim report," in *Sister Outsider: Essays and Speeches* (Berkeley, CA, Clarkson Potter/Ten Speed, 2012), 176–191.
5. *Wall Street Journal*, "This is Israel's 9/11, says Israeli ambassador to the United Nations," October 9, 2023, https://www.wsj.com/video/this-is-israel-911-says-israeli-ambassador-to-the-united-nations/EEB7D0D5-81CF-480D-A3E3-7B2FE666EE29, accessed May 12, 2025.
6. April 2025.
7. United Nations Office for the Coordination of Humanitarian Affairs, "Reported impact snapshot Gaza Strip (8 April 2025)," https://www.ochaopt.org/content/reported-impact-snapshot-gaza-strip-8-april-2025, accessed May 10, 2025.
8. Save the Children, "West Bank: Nearly half of all child killings since records began happened in the last two years," https://www.savethechildren.net/news/west-bank-nearly-half-all-child-killings-records-began-happened-last-two-years, accessed May 16, 2025.

9. World Health Organization, "People in Gaza starving, sick, dying as aid blockade continues," https://www.who.int/news/item/12-05-2025-people-in-gaza-starving--sick-and-dying-as-aid-blockade-continues, accessed May 16 2025.
10. Aya Batrawy and Anas Baba, "Gaza's hungry and malnourished children suffer under Israeli blockade," *All Things Considered*, National Public Radio, April 29, 2025, https://www.npr.org/2025/04/29/nx-s1-5380158/gazas-hungry-and-malnourished-kids-suffer-under-israeli-blockade, accessed May 16, 2025.
11. Sophia Stamatopoulou-Robbons, "The human toll: Indirect deaths from war in Gaza and the West Bank, October 7, 2023 Forward," Watson Institute for International and Public Affairs, October 7, 2024, https://watson.brown.edu/costsofwar/files/cow/imce/papers/2023/2024/Costs%20of%20War_Human%20Toll%20Since%20Oct%207.pdf, accessed May 16, 2025.
12. Condoleezza Rice, "Interview with Condoleezza Rice," interview by Wolf Blitzer, *CNN Late Edition with Wolf Blitzer*, September 8, 2022, transcript, https://transcripts.cnn.com/show/le/date/2002-09-08/segment/00, accessed May 12, 2005.
13. Walter Benjamin, "Theses on the philosophy of history," in *Illuminations* (New York, Schocken Books, 1986), 257.
14. Brandy Beard and Spencer Chrisman, "CMPD: Mother charged after 8-year-old girl dies in hot car," *WBTV News*, Charlotte, North Carolina, June 27, 2024, https://www.wbtv.com/2024/06/27/cmpd-8-year-old-dies-after-being-left-hot-car/
15. Minyvonne Burke, "Two kids sleeping in van died of carbon monoxide poisoning, not hypothermia, medical examiner says," *NBC News*, March 6, 2025, https://www.nbcnews.com/news/us-news/2-detroit-kids-sleeping-van-died-carbon-monoxide-rcna195091, accessed May 12, 2025.
16. Joseph Buczak, "Warrant sought for deaths of 2 Detroit children who died in a van, prosecutor says," *CBS News*, Detroit, March 13, 2025, https://www.cbsnews.com/

detroit/news/warrant-sought-for-deaths-of-2-detroit-children-who-died-in-van/, accessed May 12, 2025.
17. Audre Lorde, *The Cancer Journals* (New York, Penguin, 2020), 67.
18. Hebrews 11:1.

The Pluto Press Newsletter

Hello friend of Pluto!

Want to stay on top of the best radical books we publish?

Then sign up to be the first to hear about our new books, as well as special events, podcasts and videos.

You'll also get 50% off your first order with us when you sign up.

Come and join us!

Go to bit.ly/PlutoNewsletter